HOMEMADE PERFUME

Create Exquisite, Naturally Scented Products
to Fill Your Life with Botanical Aromas

ANYA McCOY
Owner of Anya's Garden Perfumes

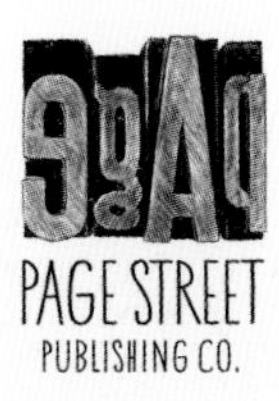

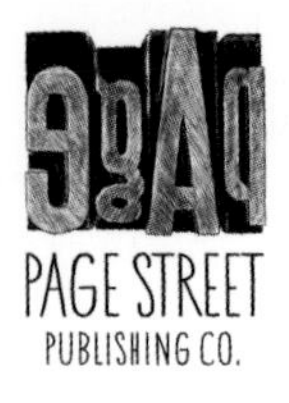

First published in 2018 by

Page Street Publishing Co.

27 Congress Street, Suite 105

Salem, MA 01970

www.pagestreetpublishing.com

Distributed by Macmillan, sales in Canada by The Canadian Manda Group.

22 21 20 19 18 1 2 3 4 5

ISBN-13: 978-1-62414-585-8

ISBN-10: 1-62414-585-X

Library of Congress Control Number: 2018932828

Cover and book design by Kylie Alexander for Page Street Publishing Co.

Photography by Jan Freire, except photos on pages 74 and 188 by Anya McCoy. Plant profile photos from pages 130–179 are from iStock, except page 167 from Shutterstock and pages 168 and 179 by Anya McCoy.

Printed and bound in the United States

Page Street Publishing protects our planet by donating to nonprofits like The Trustees, which focuses on local land conservation.

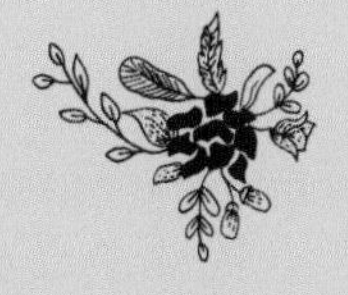

FOR ANDRINE OLSON, A SOUL SISTER ON THIS FRAGRANT PATH OF NATURAL PERFUMERY IN THE TWENTY-FIRST CENTURY

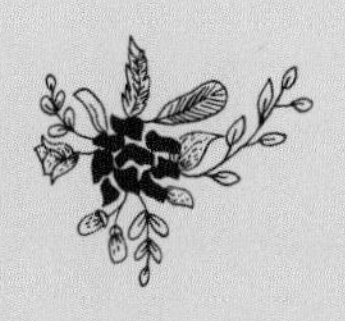

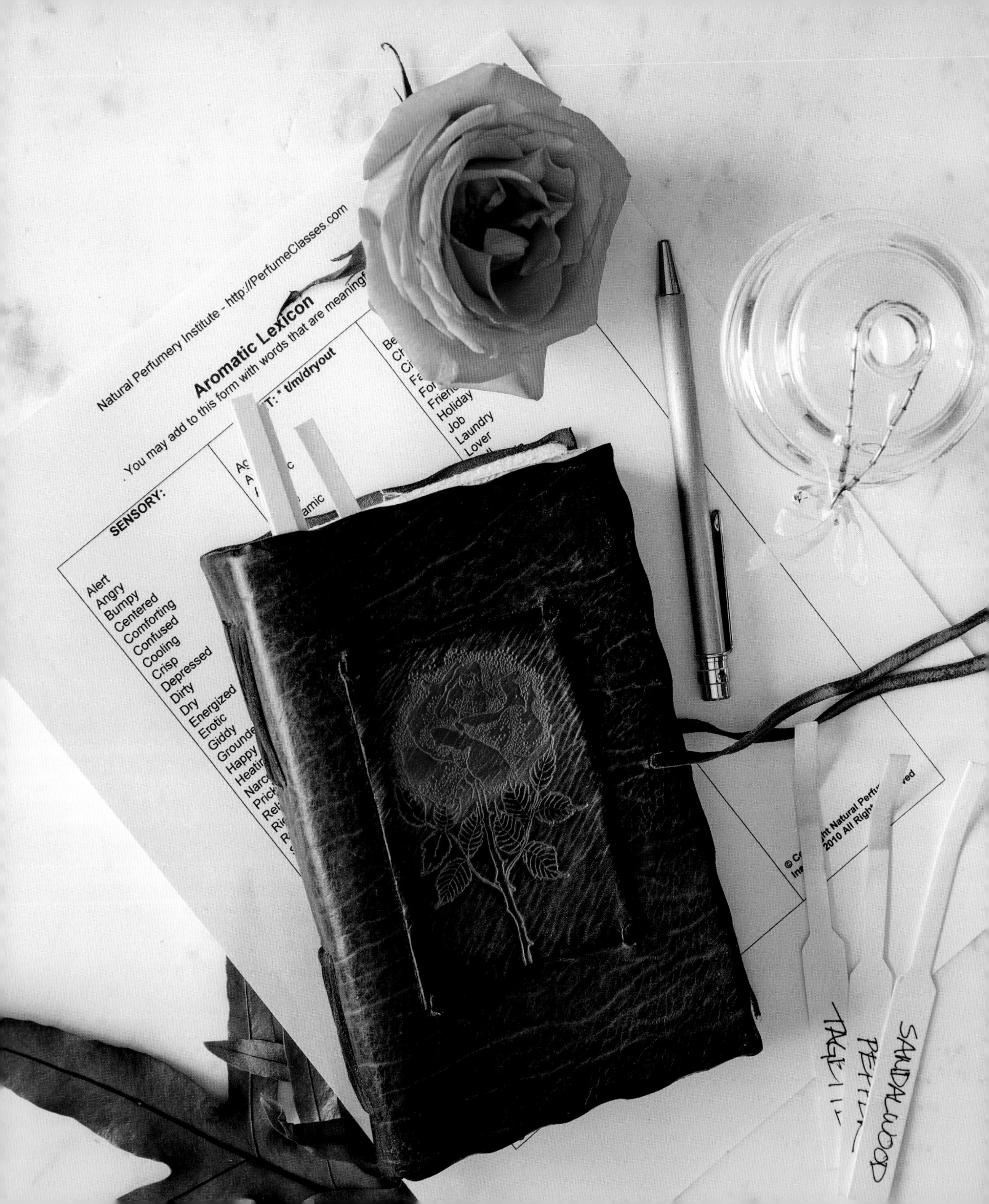
Natural Perfumery Institute - http://PerfumeClasses.com
Aromatic Lexicon
SENSORY:
Alert
Angry
Bumpy
Centered
Comforting
Confused
Cooling
Crisp
Depressed
Dirty
Dry
Energized
Erotic
Giddy
Happy
Holiday
Job
Laundry
Lover
SANDALWOOD

CONTENTS

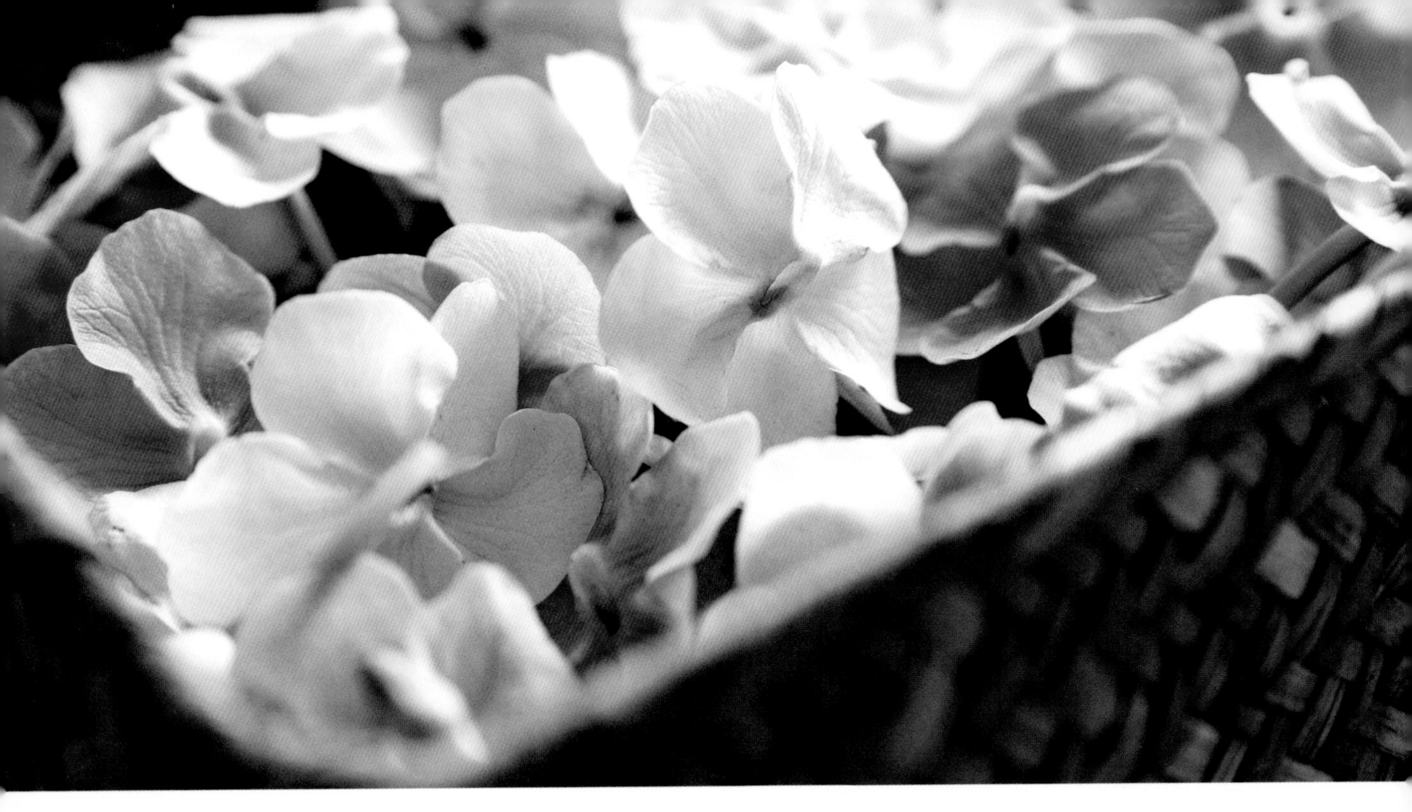

INTRODUCTION

Do you love perfume and fragrant home and body products? Are you bewitched by the fragrance of flowers, trees, and other botanicals? Do you long to capture their scents in a usable form for the body or your home in a natural, more tangible way? This book will answer all those questions for you in a fun and friendly way.

I am a dedicated "do-it-yourselfer" (DIYer) who enjoys all aspects of creating perfumes by hand, from harvesting exotic, fragrant flowers in my garden to extracting their scent, processing the extract into a usable product, bottling, and yes, even designing the labels. DIYers know the feeling of accomplishment from working a project through to completion and making creative gifts for themselves and others.

Why this, why now? Perfume making was the secret realm of the corporate perfume houses for many years, but the rise of artisan perfumery has changed all that. People like me found rare books with methods of blending perfumes, and we experimented until we hit gold—the ability to make lovely perfumes, colognes, body butters, and many more fragrant products.

As an artisan natural perfumer, aromatherapist, and herbalist, I am driven by a passion to have as much hands-on involvement as possible with the botanicals that I use in my arts. Artisan perfumers, herbalists, and home gardeners in the twenty-first century are trying their hand at capturing the scent from their plants, with varying degrees of success. Although they possess the "do-it-yourself" passion, they need a good blueprint for creating a finished product.

Over the past four decades, I have refined the lovely art of creating fragrant extracts from the plants that grow in the garden, and I've based my perfume business on it. In this book, I am passing on to you my tips and secrets for successfully creating fragrant extracts from your garden. Realistically, neither I, nor probably you, can grow enough plants to make all the scents we need for creating perfumes; sometimes it's necessary to purchase essential oils and absolutes for a truly finished fine perfume. Even body sprays, body butters, and other concoctions you'll make with directions in this book may need some final ingredients that are processed.

You may already have essential oils and absolutes on hand, and I will be recommending some for you to use. There is also the possibility you'll be very happy with homemade extracts that capture the freshness of such scents as mint, rosemary, or conifers. This book is about experimentation, creativity, and finding scents that you like and want to make, whether it's an alcohol perfume, a scented balm, a hydrosol, or a fragrant powder. *Homemade Perfume* is organized so that you can choose the method of fragrance extraction that appeals to you, read about it, and then immediately create perfumes and other scented products.

I hope that this book gives you the feeling that you are planning all of these fragrant projects with an experienced, helpful friend guiding you along the way. My biggest wish is that this book will bring you many hours of enjoyment, a sense of fulfillment, and fragrant beauties to enjoy as you become a perfume gardener who makes wonderful gifts from the earth.

You will learn how to make alcohol- and oil-based perfumes; body, room, and linen sprays; face, body, and hair vinegars; body butters; solid perfumes; and more, with your fragrant extractions and supplemental aromatics. The projects in this book are suitable for ages six and up, although children under eighteen will need supervision for most of the processes.

Enjoy, stop and smell the roses, and play with your garden's fragrant bounty. As Helen Keller said: "Smell is a potent wizard that transports you across thousands of miles and all the years you have lived." Now you will have the ability to create memorable fragrances that will have your friends and family remembering the fragrant creation you made—a living legacy of scent and delight!

Anya McCoy

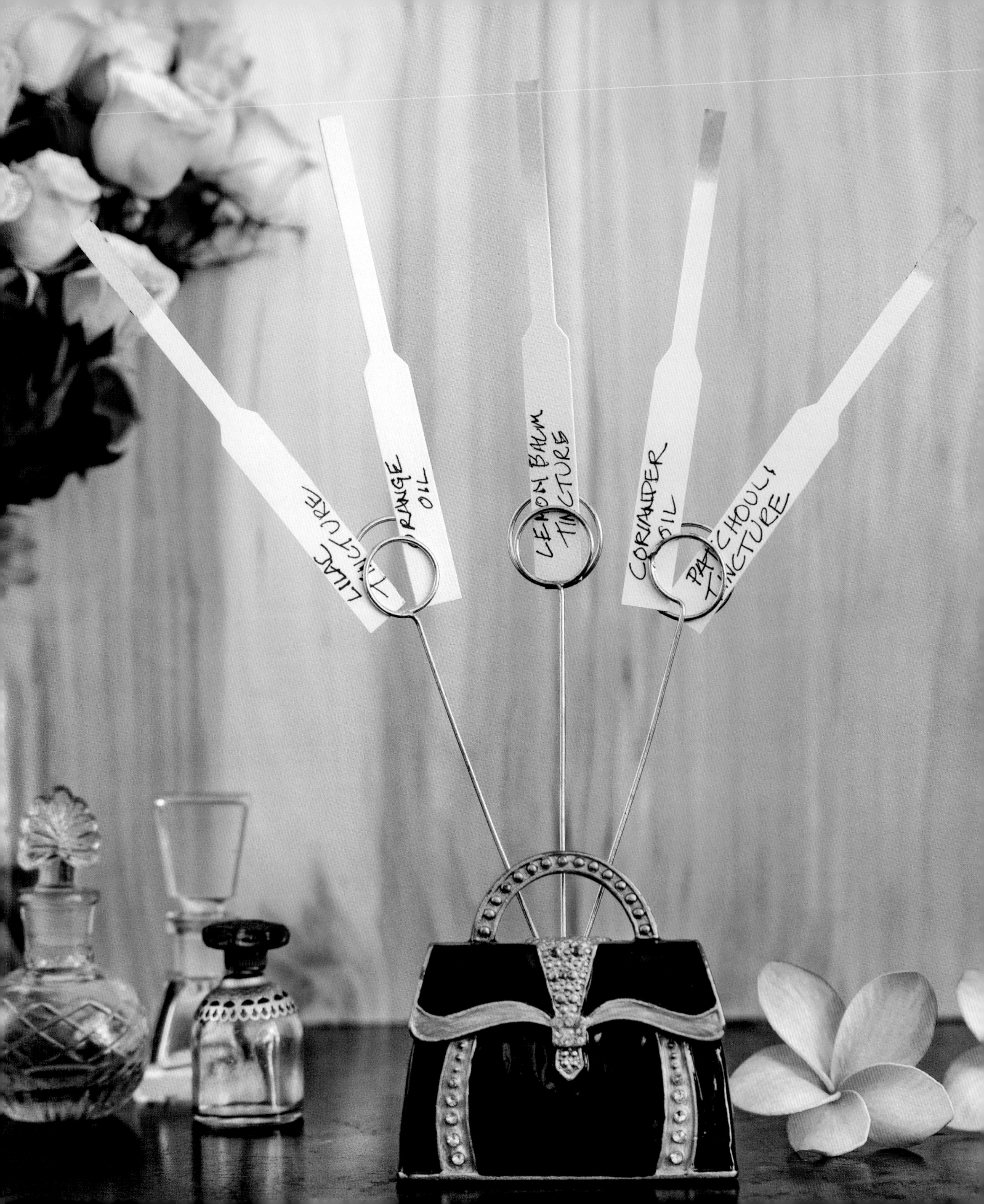
LILAC
RANGE
OIL
LEMON BALM
CTURE

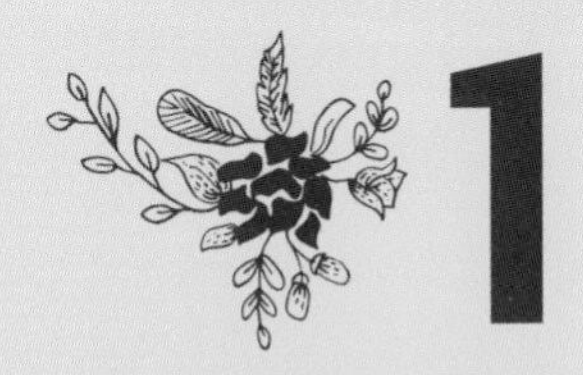

1

GETTING STARTED MAKING PERFUMES

There are easy, fun methods for extracting fragrance from plants, and in this chapter I will provide you with information that will help you get started on this journey. I wish I had had a guide like this so many years ago when I started! The trial and error of finding your way is gone—and in its place are all the details right here. You'll discover the different types of extraction, and a handy project reference so you can choose which type suits your time and expertise. I'll introduce you to perfumery terms so that you become comfortable with them and use them easily.

Don't be afraid that you'll need expensive and unattainable tools for these projects, because you'll find you may have many on hand already, or can obtain them easily. Once you get your tools and equipment together, I want to make sure you know how to clean them properly for making products you'll use on your skin or hair, or spray in the air. Safety first! I know you'll find my safety information helpful in making you confident that what you'll produce, and the time spent producing them, is up to the best standards of fragrance making.

Left: You can use creativity with objects to be used as scent strip holders. Here a decorative photo holder is perfect to securely hold the scent strips for your evaluation.

BASIC METHODS OF SCENT EXTRACTION: A BRIEF OVERVIEW

Scent extraction methods can vary from the very simple—just putting some botanicals into alcohol or oil and letting them steep—to the more complicated, such as distillation. You can pick whatever method you like, and you'll be guided step by step.

Tincturing: It's easiest to start out with tincturing, which involves a high-proof alcohol (because it pulls the most scent out of a botanical). When I started practicing herbalism years ago, tincturing involved a one-time immersion of the botanical, then straining the botanical out, and saving the liquid alcohol tincture.

Perfume tincturing is different because you have to "recharge" the tincture a number of times to fully extract the scent molecules. You can make fragrant sprays for your body, home, or linens, or create traditional perfumes with tinctures.

Infusing: Infusing botanicals in oil is another way to extract scent, and it's as easy as tincturing. You will need to recharge the oil, just as you recharge the alcohol. If you don't like using alcohol, this is the method for you. Infused fragrant oil is wonderful as a body or massage oil, scented oil perfume, or base for body butters and solid perfumes.

Distillation: The ancient art of distillation involves the use of a still, a heat source, water, and a botanical. The learning curve is a bit higher than that for tincturing, infusing, or enfleurage, but you will get two fragrant products: an essential oil and a fragrant water. The fragrant water, called a hydrosol, can also be obtained by a simple stove-top distillation method that doesn't involve a still. Instructions are provided in this book.

Enfleurage: This is a traditional French method that results in a scented solid fat or liquid oil that can be used "as is" or further processed into an extract using alcohol. The solid fat or oil enfleurage can also be used to make solid perfumes, body butters, and massage oils, similar to the uses for an infused oil. Enfleurage can also be done with powders.

PROJECT QUICK REFERENCE GUIDE

The following table is a quick guide to the extraction methods that are detailed in this book, giving their yields and the products you can make with them, as well as the level of difficulty for each method.

Project	Level of Technicality	Level of Effort	Time Required	Yield	Scented Products	Page
Tincturing	Easy	Low	Quick to moderate	Scented alcohol	Alcohol perfumes; body, room, and linen sprays	25
Infusing	Easy	Low	Moderate to long	Scented oil	Oil-based and solid perfumes; body oil; body butters	25
Distillation	Moderate to Difficult	Moderate to High	Moderate	Essential oil; hydrosol	Alcohol-based, oil-based, and solid perfumes; body, room, and linen sprays	49
Enfleurage with solid fat	Moderate	Moderate	Moderate to long	Scented pomade (shortening); alcohol extrait; absolute oil	Solid and alcohol-based perfumes; body butters	72
Enfleurage with hot oil (maceration)	Moderate	Low	Quick	Scented oil; alcohol extrait; absolute oil	Oil-based and solid perfumes; body oils; body butters	88
Enfleurage with powder	Easy	Low	Quick	Scented powder	Body powders	94
Enfleurage with vapor	Easy	Low	Quick	Scented powder	Body powders	97

HELPFUL LINGO AND TERMS TO KNOW

The following terms appear frequently and will be helpful as you start your projects:

Absolute: An aromatic substance that is produced by washing concretes (such as enfleurage pomades) in alcohol to draw out much of the scented matter, and then allowing the alcohol to evaporate or, more commonly, using vacuum distillation to remove the alcohol. Absolutes are often thick and viscous, and some may be waxy. Absolutes are regarded as the strongest aromatic product in a perfumer's palette because of their high scent concentration. You can purchase absolutes to augment your supply.

Base note: Fragrance category for the longest-lasting aromatics, which have heavy molecular weight and low volatility. They can last up to 24 hours.

Botanical: A plant or plants. Technically, of or relating to plants or plant life. In this book, when I refer to botanical it can be any part of the plant you are using for perfumery, including flowers, leaves, seeds, resin, and so on.

Concrete: A typically thick and waxy material that is extracted from raw botanicals such as jasmine, using hexane or petroleum ether as solvents, or from enfleurage pomade or oil. A concrete can be further processed into an absolute by washing it with alcohol.

Diluent: A liquid that is used to dilute aromatics such as essential oils, absolutes, resins, and others. Ethyl alcohol, jojoba oil, and even water can be used as diluents. (In modern perfumery and modern chemistry, the word dilutant is sometimes used.)

Drydown (or sometimes dryout): The persistent end experience of the perfume, dictated by the base notes. These base notes create the enduring and tenacious character of the perfume that lasts after the top and middle notes evaporate. Drydown can last up to 24 hours.

Enfleurage: A great way to extract the scent of flowers because it captures their scent at the height of its beauty. Enfleurage, whether in semi-solid fat (such as shea butter, shortening, or another waxy solid), liquid oil, or powder, has many uses for fragrant products.

Extrait: A common French term for full-strength perfume, which is 20 to 50 percent aromatics in alcohol and water. Can also be the alcohol wash from a pomade.

Maceration: The process of gently steeping delicate flowers in warmed oil for scent extraction. Maceration is a type of enfleurage. Not to be confused with hot oil infusions, which can use all types of botanical matter such as leaves and roots, maceration is done only with flowers.

Middle note: Fragrance category for the aromatics that make up the middle of a perfume blend. Often apparent at the opening of the perfume, but the aromatics in this category are less volatile (evaporative) than top notes, becoming most noticeable after the top-note drydown—about fifteen to twenty minutes after applying. Middle notes typically last for two to eight hours.

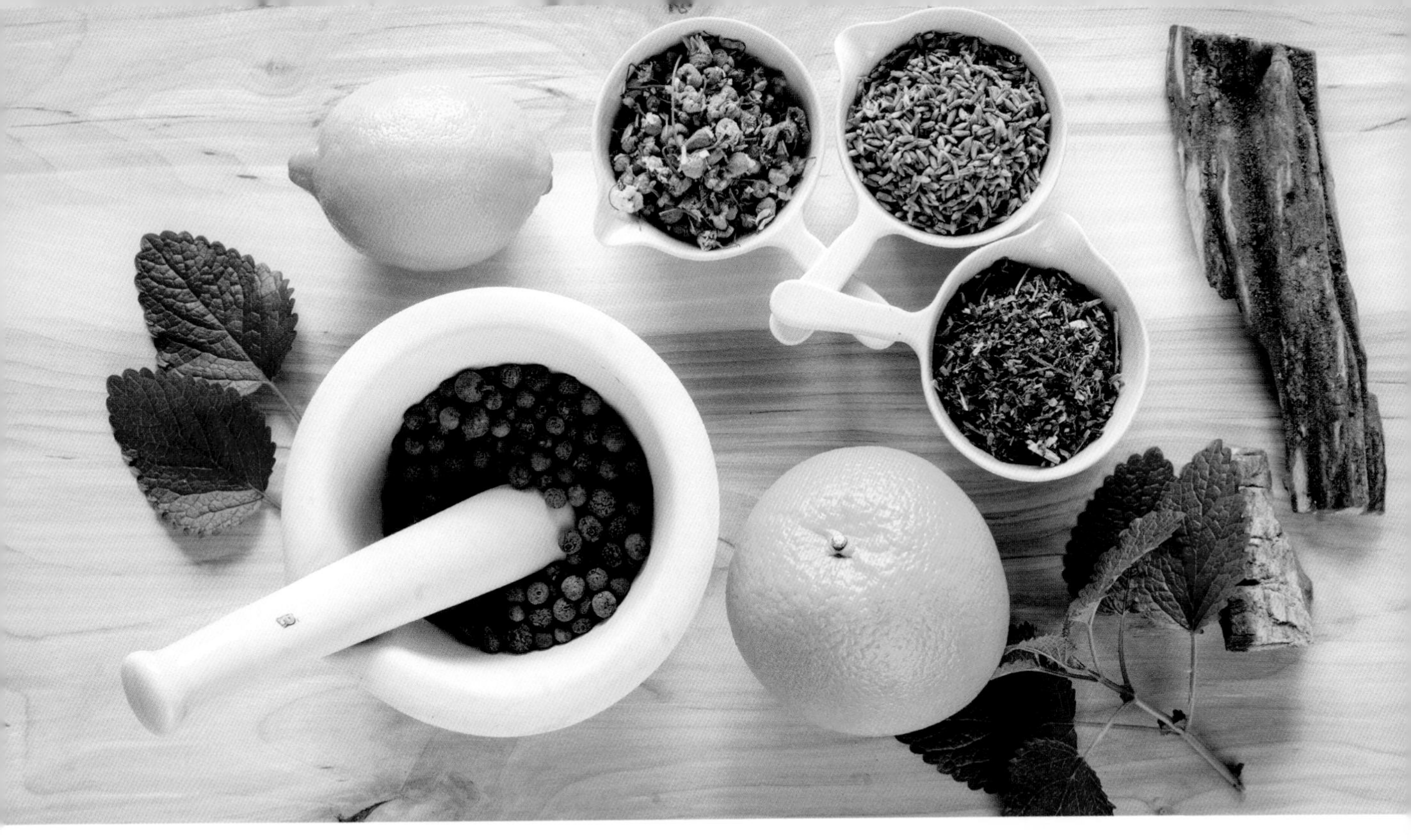

Many fragrant plant parts used in perfumery are everyday botanicals that you are familiar with and can easily grow or obtain. Plant parts used in perfume, from left to right: leaves (e.g., mint), seeds (e.g., allspice berries), flowers (e.g., chamomile, lavender), fermented leaves (patchouli), citrus peels (e.g., orange), and wood (e.g., palo santo).

Pomade: The product of the first step in historical enfleurage, when flowers are placed upon fat to extract the scent. Also called pommade.

Recharge: To replace the botanical in your tincture, infusion, or enfleurage as many times as you want until the scent strength satisfies you.

Solvent: A substance used for dissolving another substance. Alcohol is the most universal solvent in perfumery; water is the most universal solvent in nature. Aromatics can also be solvents, capable of dissolving each other, or dissolving varnish from a wood surface, marring a plastic surface, and performing other destructive actions.

Spent: When flowers and leaves are immersed in a liquid solvent, after a period of time they lose their structure and become soft and floppy. Flowers may even become translucent. This is known as the spent condition, meaning they have given up their freshness and scent to the solvent.

Top note: The introductory, most volatile note in a perfume. Top notes are low in molecular weight, and thus, they vaporize in a short time, typically from two to twenty minutes. Aromatics such as citrus and spices are top notes.

ESSENTIAL TOOLS AND MATERIALS

Convenient and affordable—that's my aim when looking for tools to extract the scent from botanicals and when creating perfumes! You may already have many of the necessary tools around your house, like jars with lids, funnels, pots for boiling jars and bottles to sterilize them, spoons, and bowls. You may also have oils and waxes that are used in extraction processes. High-proof alcohol is needed, and you may have to purchase that. Internet sales sites are good sources for some of the items, especially laboratory glassware and gadgets.

Fragrant Plants

If you have a garden with fragrant plants, you are ready to begin working. If not, a list of suggested plants appears in Chapter 6, and suppliers for plants and seeds are provided in Appendix 3.

Bottles and Jars

You will use these for preparing tinctures, infusions, and hot oil enfleurage, and for storing some of your materials and finished products. Glass is best for storing tinctures and essential oils because it is nonreactive. You will probably want more decorative bottles and jars when you make fragrant products for gift giving. Most of the bottle and jar suppliers listed in Appendix 3 carry a selection of decorative glassware and plastic jars. For onetime product packaging, you might have an item in your house that you can use. You can also find bottles and jars in thrift or antique stores and at garage sales.

Everyday Glass Jars

Use these for processing and storage. For durability, I choose to make and store my extracts in canning jars. The thick glass, the rubber-rimmed lids, and the screw-on rings provide a sturdy, easy-to-store, airtight container. It's also easy to replace any of the separate parts. I tend to use three jar sizes: 8, 16, and 32 ounces (237, 473, and 946 ml). It's also a nice aesthetic to have matching jars for your apothecary.

Plastic Jars

Many cosmetics suppliers and bottle-supply houses carry both utilitarian and more decorative plastic jars. You may wish to store carrier oils (also called fixed oils, or base oils), waxes, and other nonreactive materials in plastic jars. Sometimes the jars that the materials arrive in from the supplier are sufficient.

NOTE: Never use plastic containers for tincturing or making perfumes. The alcohol can dissolve plastic, causing plastic molecules to leach into the tincture. Some essential oils can do the same. Additionally, the scent of your products will permeate the plastic, giving it a permanent odor.

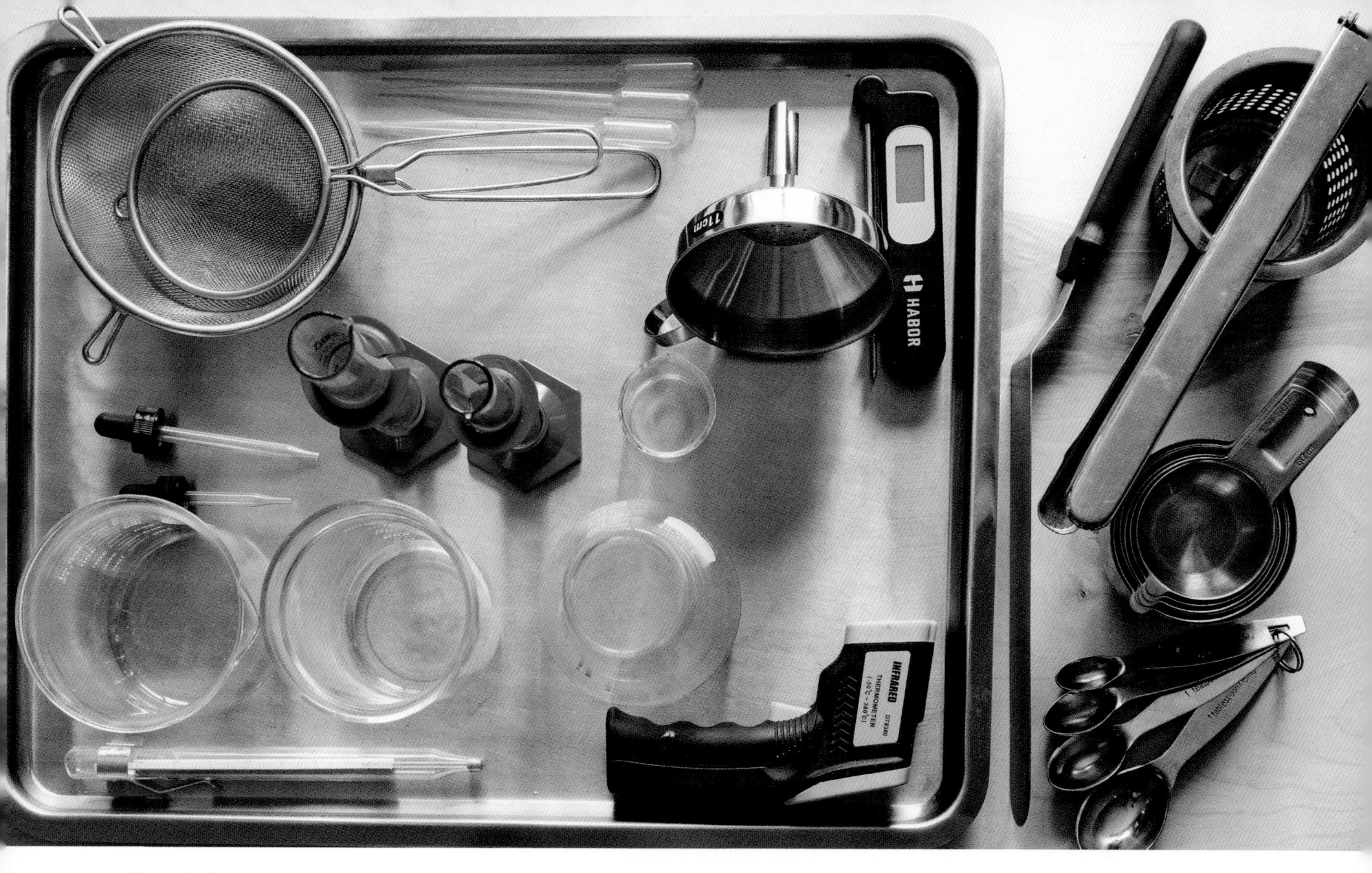

From left to right, at top: stainless steel strainers, stainless steel funnels, instant-read thermometer. Middle row: droppers, graduated cylinders, small beaker. Bottom: large beakers, candy thermometer, infra-red thermometer. Right side: offset spatula, potato ricer, stainless steel measuring cups and spoons.

Measuring Cups, Measuring Spoons, and Volumetric Beakers

Measuring cups and spoons provide an easy way to determine the volume of both solid and liquid materials for simple projects that do not require precision, such as those involving tinctures and infusions. I recommend nonreactive stainless steel or glass for perfumery work.

Volumetric beakers are wide, cylindrical glass containers with precise volumetric markings on the sides, in increments of 25 milliliters to 1,000 milliliters, depending on the size. You may find regular-weight beakers useful in making some products when precise measurements are needed. However, I recommend lightweight beakers, usually called borosilicate beakers, if you're weighing materials. They come in various sizes, typically from 50 milliliters to 1,000 milliliters. I recommend various sizes, from 25 to 50 milliliters for beginners. You can always add to the set of beakers later. When you purchase beakers, you may want to get watch glass covers for them as well. These are useful for protecting your beakers from dust and foreign matter and are also helpful when you're using the beakers to evaporate the alcohol from extraits.

Graduated cylinders are narrow, cylindrical glass containers with more defined, detailed volumetric markings on the side, which can go to as low as 1⁄10 milliliter.

Pipettes and Droppers

A pipette, or pipete, is typically a narrow tube of plastic or glass that is used to measure specific amounts of liquids or to withdraw a liquid from a container easily. I recommend the pipettes that have a rubber bulb on the end opposite the liquid uptake. The bulb is squeezed to create a slight vacuum, drawing the liquid into the pipette tube. Manual pipettes are inexpensive. You can purchase either glass or plastic pipettes, reusable or disposable. They are easily cleaned by washing them in hot, soapy water.

Droppers are similar to pipettes, with slight differences. They are typically wider than pipettes. The dropper may have a screw-top cap attached and can be affixed to a bottle with a matching thread pattern. I recommend getting some glass bottles with matching dropper tops to hold your essential oils or extraits. That way, your liquid is stored in a container with a dropper, making it easy to transfer the liquid or to count drops. Tip: Monprene bulbs for droppers are more resistant to degradation than rubber bulbs.

Strainers

Several options are available for separating your plant matter from the solvent. You will likely need a number of these items in several different sizes.

Cloth strainers are most typically cheesecloth or muslin. These are nice because they can be stretched across a colander or other apparatus that allows the plant material to be placed inside the cheesecloth or muslin and strained.

I prefer stainless steel strainers because they are nonreactive and come in several sizes.

Herb presses and potato ricers make it easy to squeeze the solvent from the plant material. Metal potato ricers are inexpensive and easy to find. I recommend lining the bottom with gauze or a cheesecloth to filter smaller bits of plant material from the tincture.

Filter Papers

When you're creating your tinctures, oils, and perfumes, it's important to remove even the smallest particles from them so that they're as clear as possible. This is achieved by pouring them through paper filters, such as unbleached coffee filters or laboratory filters (available from laboratory-supply companies).

If you use coffee filters, it's best to rinse them in water and hang them to dry before using them. Some contain stiffening agents, or they may have a paper smell that could transfer to your extrait. Lab filter papers come in various pore sizes; the smaller the pore, the more efficient the filter. The flat, round papers are sized by diameter in inches or centimeters. Choose the diameter by measuring across the widest part of your funnel. For a 6-inch (150-mm) funnel, you need either 150-millimeter (it will not quite reach the top edge of the funnel) or 180-millimeter paper, which will reach higher than the funnel top.

Trays

Nonreactive trays made of either enamel or stainless steel will protect your work surfaces. Because alcohol is a powerful solvent, it can ruin a table's finish, and an oil spill creates a mess; that's why I prefer to do my work on trays. Search eBay and thrift stores for stainless steel dental trays, or the enameled trays called butcher trays, that are at least 12 by 18 inches (30 by 46 cm).

For enfleurage of big flowers, I use the steam table pans with lids that you see in cafeterias and at catered events. They vary from about 2.5 inches (6 cm) to 4 inches (10 cm) deep. The lids for these pans provide a good seal. If you want a tighter seal, you can use clothespins or office clamps.

Thermometers

To help you monitor the heat when you're making a hot extraction, it's a good idea to use some sort of thermometer. The following options work well for making perfume extractions:

- **Candy or fat thermometers** are immersed in liquids for reading.
- **Instant-read thermometers** can also be immersed in liquid.
- **Infrared "gun" thermometers** are used to read surface heat only and are not immersible in liquid.

Labels

Labels are crucial for keeping all of your botanicals, bottles, and bits and pieces of "stuff" identifiable and organized. You won't be terribly happy if you find an unlabeled jar in the back of a cabinet sometime after making it and can't figure out what it is. Many labels that are sold in office-supply stores are not suitable for glass jars or plastic containers because they're made for paper, and they may not adhere well to another type of surface. Before buying labels for this purpose, confirm with the seller that they will adhere to glass, metal, plastic, and paper. You may want to print on higher-quality labels for your products that you plan to give as gifts, or if you expand your art into a profession.

Scent Strips and Holders

These are paper strips used for sampling aromatics and any liquid extracts that you make, as well as essential oils and absolutes. The premade ones are available online from various sources, usually costing about $6 for a pack of 100. I recommend the paddle-style scent strips that have a narrow tip for dipping into the bottle, and a broader end where you can write the information about the aromatic that you are studying.

You can make your own scent strips from watercolor paper. Buy some inexpensive, acid-free paper with a pressed surface, of at least 120-pound (54-kg) weight. Cut the paper into strips about 7 inches (18 cm) long by 1 inch (2.5 cm) wide. You can trim one end much thinner if you need to fit it into narrow-necked bottles.

You will also need something to hold the scent strips while you evaluate aromatics. You can use photo holders or memo holders. You can also place scent strips upright in small beakers, with the aromatic end sticking up while you assess the scent.

NOTE: Do not store your scent strips near your aromatics. They can absorb the scents that escape into the air from the bottles, even when the bottles are tightly closed. You may wish to store them in a glass jar with a tight-fitting lid.

Heating Units

Several of the processes in this book call for heating the solvent and plant material. The following are some common options available to accomplish this:

- **Slow cookers** are inexpensive and easily obtained. One limitation for infusions may be that slow cookers become too hot, even on the lowest setting.
- **Double boilers** (sometimes called a bain-marie) apply gentle heat from steam. Water is heated in a vessel, and another vessel is placed on top of it, containing the plant material and a solvent, which is typically oil. The upper pot does not touch the water below, and thus avoids scorching the plant material. If you don't own a double boiler, you can easily improvise one using a nonreactive pot, such as stainless steel, heat-proof glass, or enamel, and a tempered glass or stainless steel bowl that will fit into the pot/saucepan but will not submerge in the water. The top bowl that holds the botanical is covered with a tight-fitting lid.
- **Hot plates** are useful for individual heating jobs and are handy because you can use them outside, not tying you to the kitchen.
- **Cup warmers** are used for heating a beaker or a small bowl or jar. Like hot plates, they can be used indoors or outside, but they don't get as hot.
- **Stove tops**, either electric, gas, induction, or another system, can be used for making infusions and just about any process that calls for heat. Some stove tops have special warming areas that produce a lower heat than that of the regular burners.

Distillation Systems

Several different types of distillation systems are available in many sizes. Even though the cost of distillation systems has come down recently, they are still the most expensive apparatus mentioned in this book. You can choose from copper alembics that are best suited for making hydrosols, or glass or stainless steel distilling units that extract essential oils well. Or you can buy the parts and build a system yourself.

SAFELY CLEANING EQUIPMENT FOR PROJECTS

Many people use the terms sanitize, disinfect, and sterilize interchangeably, but this is incorrect. It's incredibly important that you properly clean all of the tools and containers for each project so that you prevent contamination, which would not only spoil your hard work but can also be a safety hazard.

In this section I'll give you the steps to properly clean your equipment depending on what you're using it for. The first level, sanitization, removes a lot of the surface germs, but it is not sufficient to prevent the spread of the microbes in some of your products. After sanitizing, you need to disinfect the equipment, which will remove almost 100 percent of microbes. This is suitable for most surfaces and objects you will be using. Sterilization of equipment is needed for hydrosols, but it can also be your chosen method if you want to ensure that all of the microbes are killed or deactivated.

Your equipment and containers, and the degree of cleanliness they require, play an important role in the success of your extracts and bottling. Yes, the plant material that you place in these containers cannot be sanitized, disinfected, or sterilized before processing, but most of the processes to refine the scented products will destroy microbes. After years of processing flowers, leaves, and other plant parts, I have only had some failures with oil infusions, which is why I give you specific, cautionary instructions when making infusions.

Sanitize: Make Everything Basically Clean

The first thing you need to do before using any jar, bottle, tray, beaker, stirring implement, or other tool is make your hands sanitary. This is accomplished by vigorously washing with soap and hot water for 20 to 30 seconds. Then you need to sanitize your tools because you don't know what dust, chemical, or other possible contaminant may be on the surface or inside a jar or bottle.

Wash the objects in hot, soapy water and rinse with hot water. Place jars or bottles upside down on a clean towel or cloth to dry. If you have a dishwasher, all the better. Make sure the objects are suitable for the dishwasher, and run a cycle with minimal detergent. The super-hot water will do most of the work. Use the dry cycle, and when you remove the objects, take care to protect them from dust or other contaminants before use.

You may use chlorine bleach to sanitize around the house, but I do not recommend its use for perfumery because of potential toxic effects and the lingering smell. However, if you wish, 1 tablespoon (15 ml) of bleach in 1 gallon (3.8 L) of water will sanitize.

Disinfect: Remove Most Microbes

The easiest way to disinfect your objects is to wash them with 151-proof alcohol. Pour a small amount of the alcohol into a bottle or jar, place the cap or lid on the bottle or jar, and gently shake the vessel for a minute to coat and cover the inside. Depending on the size of the object, anywhere from a tablespoon to a few ounces may be needed. For objects like stirrers and beakers, you may pour the alcohol from one container or object to another, and also pour over stirrers, spoons, and other tools to coat them. Allow 10 minutes before use so the alcohol can work.

If you wish to use bleach, ¼ cup (60 ml) per 1 gallon (3.8 L) of water is used, and the 10-minute waiting period is the minimum time needed.

Protect the objects from recontamination after disinfection.

Sterilize: Kill or Deactivate All Microbes

The sterilization process is easily accomplished by boiling an object for 20 minutes. This is mandatory for any object that comes in touch with hydrosols as soon as the hydrosol leaves the still or stove top. Another method of sterilization is provided by a UV (ultraviolet) unit, such as the type used by manicurists and tattoo artists. There are units with a shelf, so you have two levels to work with. Place glass jars and bottles on the top shelf, and lids and caps on the lower shelf, facing up, so that the UV light passing through the glass can reach them. Most units come with a timer, and 15 minutes is typical for this type of sterilization.

SAFETY CONSIDERATIONS

Safety first, that's my motto. Always work in a well-ventilated space, whether you're making simple tinctures or infusions, or distilling. Aromatic molecules can be a bit strong in an enclosed space, so if you feel the need, open a window, turn on a fan, or take a step outside for some fresh air.

Essential oils are very concentrated, so if you spill some on your skin or a surface, wash well with water immediately. They might cause a skin rash or, on a surface, remove the varnish or damage the item.

The most important safety issue involves working with alcohol. Alcohol is flammable, so adult supervision is needed when children are working on a project.

When working with heated alcohol, good ventilation is imperative to prevent vapors from accumulating and increasing explosion risk. The alcohol must be gently warmed, never hot or scalding; keep it in the range of 86 to 104°F (30 to 40°C).

These are important factors for two reasons. First, the higher the temperature, the greater the chance of alcohol or fumes igniting. Second, higher temperatures cause evaporation, diffusing alcohol and aromatics into the air and wasting some of the precious scent that you worked hard to extract.

Because of these safety issues, I debated for several years whether or not to use heat with alcohol. Once I got up the nerve to try it, I put many controls in place, such as maintaining good ventilation; using an electrical heat source only, with no open flame nearby; and focusing with laser-like obsession on every step of what I'm doing (something I'm not known for!). Needless to say, I'm delighted with the ease of working with alcohol and heat.

A final word on alcohol safety: Because it's the perfect solvent for working with aromatic extracts, high-proof alcohol is a blessing. But never forget that its same power as a solvent can damage furniture, cause a fire, and do bodily harm. Treat it as you would any other highly volatile substance: with caution and respect.

Now you're ready to start having fun with aromatic botanicals! You can proceed with the confidence that you have some basic knowledge of the tools and materials needed, as well as the safety factors that must be followed.

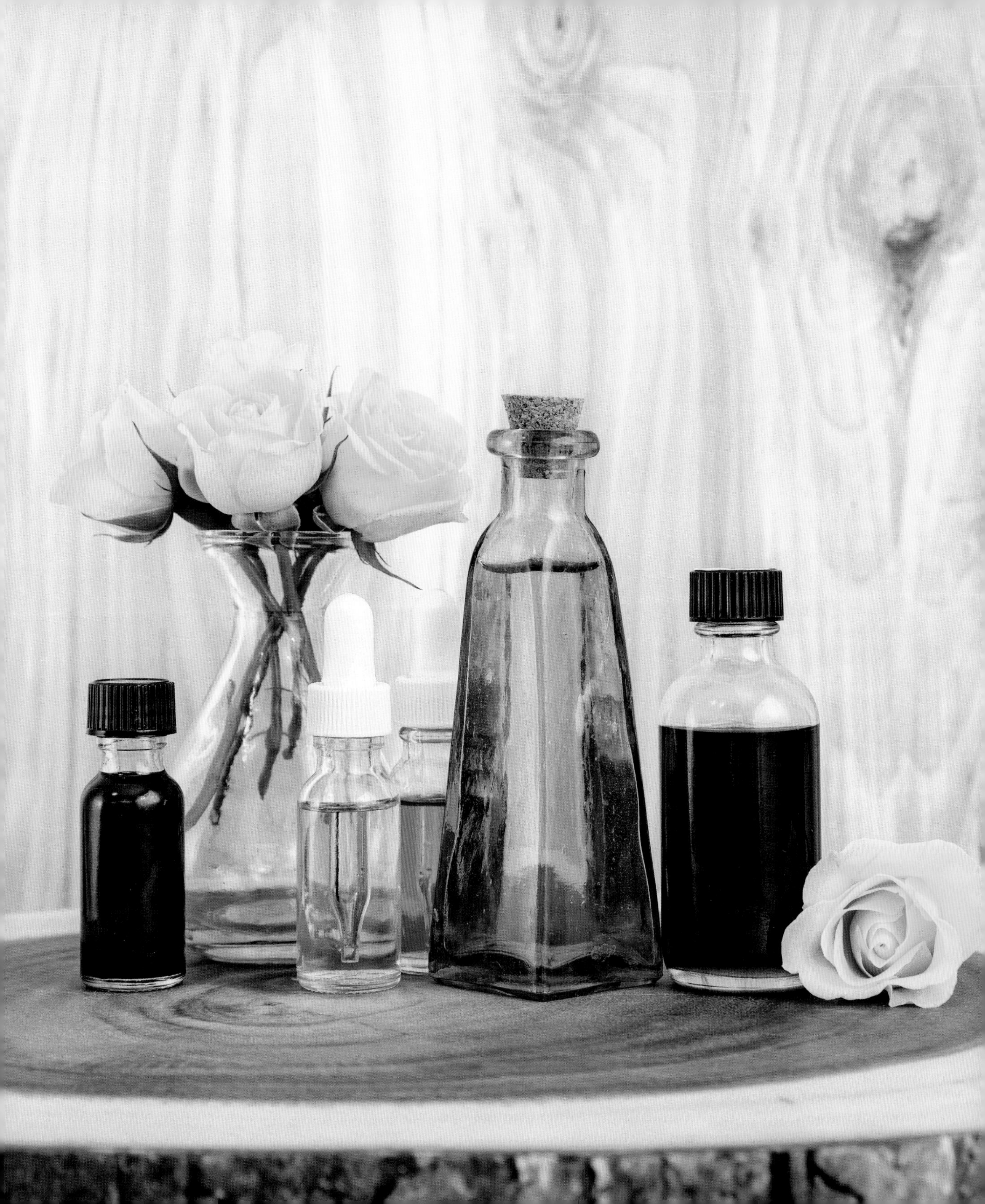

2

TINCTURES AND INFUSIONS

Tincturing and infusing are two of the oldest methods for extracting useful elements from plant materials. Infusion is the older of the two, because expressed oils and fats were available thousands of years before high-proof alcohols. The only method that is older than these two is burning fragrant materials in fires or censers. These practices are medicinal and enjoyable at the same time.

Left: There is something so satisfying in extracting fragrance from plants. You'll have an array of fabulous creations to make your perfumes, body oils, body butters, and more. Shown from left to right: absolute oil, tinctures in dropper bottles, infused oil, and essential oil.

INTRODUCTION TO TINCTURING AND INFUSING

Tincturing and its cousin infusing are the quickest, easiest ways to extract scent from plants. What do I mean by easy? At its most basic level, all you need to make a tincture is alcohol, glass jars, cheesecloth, and the fresh or dried plant material. You place the botanicals in 190-proof alcohol, which is a powerful solvent that causes the scent molecules to dissolve into it.

I've added vinegar as a solvent for special skin-care and hair-care tinctures. Since ancient times, fragrant botanicals such as rose, rosemary, and chamomile have been infused in vinegar for beauty purposes. Once the scent strength is reached, you dilute the vinegar with distilled water. I love the fragrant, healthy results on my face, body, and hair, and I know you will, too.

Perfumers who grow plants that are not extracted by the mainstream fragrance industry can create unique additions to their stock by tincturing them. These plants include lilac, honeysuckle, rare jasmines, and certain herbs, as well as other materials, such as scented leaves, woods, roots, and barks. In my experience, tincturing fresh, slightly wilted flowers often captures the most volatile, fleeting top notes of the flower, along with most of the other scent molecules.

All nonpoisonous, nonirritating, nonallergenic plant parts can be tinctured. Flowers take the least amount of time, while harder, denser materials—roots, branches, bark, seeds, and thick leaves—take more time. Each plant brief in Chapter 6 gives approximate times for tincturing the particular plant material.

All About Infusing

Infusing is similar to tincturing, but instead of alcohol, the solvent is now an oil with little scent, such as moringa, coconut, argan, grapeseed, or light olive oil, or a liquid wax, such as jojoba oil. I felt absolute delight when, years ago, I made my first oil-based infusion. I was working with herbs for healing, but then I quickly discovered how easy it is to make scented oils for perfumery purposes. Calendula flowers, a lovely skin-soothing botanical, gave up a spicy, green scent, but dried rosebuds were ambrosia. I was hooked! What fun to have a quick and easy way to capture plant scent. I know you'll enjoy this, too, and find many ways to use the oil.

There are several processes for infusing botanicals, varying from the oldest and least technical methods to the latest methods using modern technology to assist in the procedure. You can make cold or hot infusions, basing your decision on the plant you choose and your goal. Cold infusion works well with flowers and delicate leaves. Because heat helps to draw the scent from within plant cells, hot infusion works best with tougher, harder materials such as thicker leaves, woods, and roots.

This extraction method yields a beautifully fragrant product that can be used as an oil perfume applied directly to skin or hair. Additionally, the scented oil combines well with a solid wax, such as beeswax, to make solid perfumes and is also used in body-care products.

We've all experienced oil that turns bad, even in the kitchen for cooking purposes, and it is painful to have to toss an infused oil that you spent a lot of time and effort on. It helps to refrigerate these oils to slow down their expiration.

For infusions, it's important to use oils that have a long shelf life, such as moringa oil or jojoba oil, unless you plan to make products that will be used within a year. For products with a shorter shelf life, you can use almond, grapeseed, or any other oil you like.

Common Ground between Tincturing and Infusing

Tincturing and infusing are two of the quickest, easiest ways to extract the scent from plants, and they require little equipment besides the appropriate liquid, a few airtight containers, and a little time. With either method, you place the plant material in a jar and complete the following steps:

1. Cover it with the solvent of choice.
2. After the designated extraction time, according to the solvent and the plant, strain the tincture or infusion.
3. Recharge the original solvent with the botanical, repeating the timing and straining schedules, until the solvent is saturated with scent, or until you reach the desired scent strength.

PREPARING BOTANICALS FOR TINCTURING OR INFUSING

I love it if you think of yourself as a perfume gardener, either growing the botanicals yourself or getting some from friends or family members who have an excess of fragrant plants. However, you can also purchase them, as I do sometimes with gardenias since I don't grow many of them. I don't mind paying a little to get a great reward in the perfume department!

Before putting your botanicals to macerate in any solvent, you may need to prepare them in some way. The quality of your end products is directly affected by the care with which you treat the fresh plant material. It's best to harvest botanicals when they're free from moisture, such as rain or morning dew. See specific plant briefs in Chapter 6 for information on what time of day to harvest, if applicable.

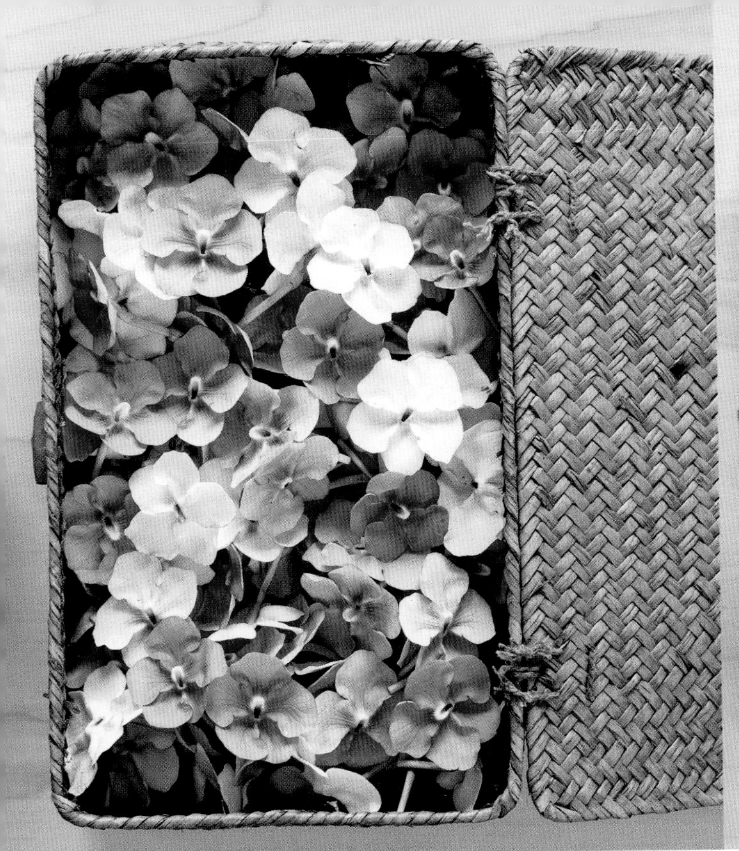

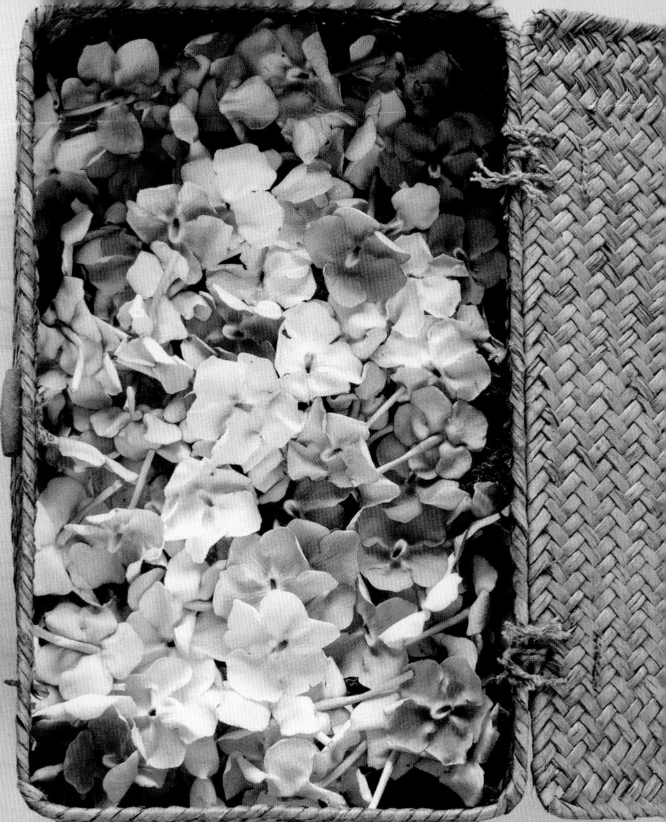

If you put freshly-picked flowers (shown on left) into alcohol or oil, the water content may seep into the liquid and that is something you don't want. Follow the instructions on how to slightly wilt the flowers (shown on right) to allow a lot of the water to evaporate before you process the blooms, and that will avoid water problems in your extract.

Fresh plants must be processed as quickly as possible after harvesting. They require slight wilting before infusing or tincturing.

To wilt your fresh botanicals, simply spread a towel, cheesecloth, or other porous material over a drying rack (an oven or cooling rack works), and lay your plant materials on them.

> **TIP:** Don't wilt delicate flowers for more than an hour, or they can lose their top notes. Let your nose be your guide on the scent, and pay close attention to the look and feel of the botanical during wilting. You want it to look slightly softer, but not distressed or browning. It shouldn't feel sticky or slippery either.

Dried botanicals, such as leaves or flower petals, might not need any preparation before you place them in the solvent. Others, such as bark or seeds, may need to be broken up, or even ground in order to expose more of the botanical to the solvent.

Caution with Fresh Botanicals in Infusions

There is one important caveat when you're using fresh botanicals for infusions: The water content of plants causes them to decay rapidly because an oil solvent does not have the sterilization properties of an alcohol solvent. You can do several things to help protect your infusions from spoilage:

- Make sure to wilt your plant matter, as described previously, and observe the times provided in the Levels Method Timetable on page 32. This step can minimize the amount of water released into the infusion and prevent it from spoiling.
- While your botanical is infusing, do not shake the jar because that will create air bubbles, which can allow microbial growth in the solvent.
- If you see that the flowers or leaves are limp and spent, or have turned translucent, strain them from the solvent, return the solvent to the jar, and recharge it with more of the same plant (you'll learn more about recharging an infusion on page 33).
- You must check the jar daily until the infusion is complete in order to ensure that the plant material and any water that leaches from it have not begun to decay or produce bacteria.
- If water leaches from the plant material, it appears as a separate layer at the bottom of the jar. If you notice water at the bottom of your infusion, you must carefully decant the oil layer and plant material into another sterile jar, leaving the water layer undisturbed. Because microbes can grow in water, you risk ruining an infusion if any water mixes with the oil when you're straining or decanting it.
- I sometimes use pipettes to remove as much water as possible from the bottom of the infusion before I pour the oil or remove any of the botanical from it. The goal is to obtain a clean decant. If you are using dried materials, water isn't an issue.
- To decant, carefully pour off the oil, stopping before you reach the water layer. Discard the remaining water and oil portion. You'll sacrifice a little of your oil with the intent of lessening the possibility of bringing over some water with it. If you wish, use that oil to rub on your hand, arm, or hair so it isn't totally wasted.

THE SIMPLERS' MEASURING METHOD

In the perfume world, several methods are employed for measuring and combining plant materials and solvents. However, for simplicity, this book mainly uses only one method: the simplers' method. With its roots in home-based herbalism from centuries past, this is the oldest and easiest method for combining botanicals and solvents for extraction. In those times, the term herbal simple was given to remedies measured by volume and derived from a single plant. Called "simplers," the people who made these remedies were predominantly women. Other methods require precise weighing and measuring and are most often used by professional perfumers.

You will learn to blend your perfumes in Chapter 5, using the volumetric method, which is the easiest way to measure the various liquids. Also known as volume/volume, or v/v, measuring, this method uses percent as its basis. Making solutions to a specific volume percent concentration typically requires volumetric beakers and graduated cylinders. You may need to measure as little as 1 milliliter of a highly concentrated tincture or extrait for your perfumes, so the precise volumetric beakers will be helpful.

If you need to calculate percentages and ratios for any reason, see Appendix 3 for links to online calculators.

TINCTURING AND INFUSING TIMES

I started a natural perfumery group on Yahoo in 2002, and one of the perennially popular topics in the Yahoo Natural Perfumery group is tincturing and infusing plant materials. As the "list mom," I watched discussions go back and forth on how long to allow the botanical to remain in the solvent before removing it. Some people believe that plants should remain in the solvent until the petals or leaves turn translucent, while others have varied opinions, including only briefly dipping them in the alcohol for a few seconds or, conversely, leaving them in for weeks. Because water invites bacteria into the solvent, the latter option is questionable, especially with large, thick-petaled flowers, such as magnolias and gardenias, because they have a higher water content than thinner-petaled flowers and leaves.

In herbalism, the botanical is left in the jar to macerate with the solvent for weeks in order to extract more healing molecules from the herb. However, for tincturing, herbalists typically use a lower-proof alcohol for the solvent, anywhere from 40 proof to 150 proof. The water that makes up the rest of the solvent acts as a solvent for the water-soluble parts of the botanical.

For perfumery, on the other hand, the botanical is extracted into a higher-proof alcohol, and the plant matter is left in the solvent for as short a time as possible to extract the scent, while extracting as little water as possible. I have found that up to 24 hours is sufficient. Because alcohol is hygroscopic, meaning it draws water from the plant, excessive maceration dilutes the alcohol percentage, making the extraction weaker and more susceptible to spoilage or cloudiness.

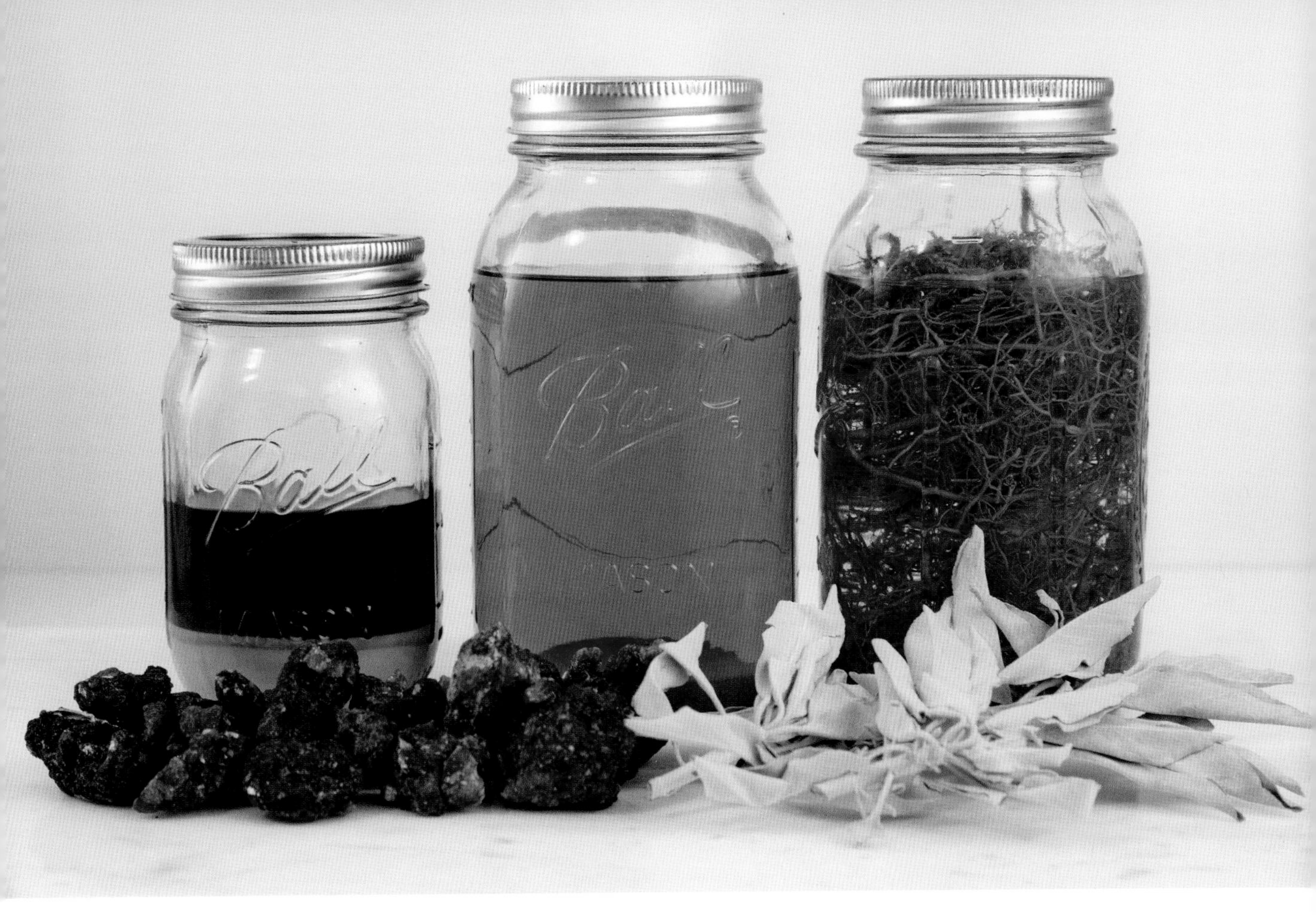

Some botanicals, especially dried, powdered ones, separate into layers with your extraction solvent, so frequent shaking of the jar is needed. Shown from left to right, back: orris powder tincture (unfiltered), jasmine tincture (filtered), and vetiver root infusion (unfiltered); front: opoponax resin and white sage.

After decades of hands-on experimentation, and many failures and successes with tincturing and infusing, I developed a quick-reference, level-based method for extraction times, where the levels delineate the maceration time ranges that various types of plants require. The Levels Method Timetable on page 32 lists the type of plant material, the extraction method, and the length of maceration time the botanical needs for successful extraction. This table is the companion to the tables provided for each plant listed in Chapter 6.

With infusions, the oils extract scent more slowly than alcohol does, so you will see different times for tincturing and infusing for the same types of botanicals.

The maceration times in this table are merely guidelines. Feel free to experiment and play with them to determine more precise times for the specific botanicals you're working with.

To reduce the amount of water released into the solvent, remember to subject your plant matter to a wilting stage (see page 28).

LEVELS METHOD TIMETABLE

Level 1: Tincturing	Level 1: Infusing
Time: Up to 24 hours **Plant Type:** Fragile flowers, such as jasmine, gardenias, violets, and roses. Thinner, more delicate leaves, such as mint, scented geraniums, and dried herbs. Slightly wilt in a cool, dry place; spread in a single layer for an hour or so. Wilt thick-petaled flowers, such as gardenias or magnolias, for a few hours before tincturing. Leave these botanicals in the alcohol for no longer than 24 hours, which is sufficient time to extract the scent molecules. Longer maceration pulls unwanted water from the plant, diluting your tincture.	**Time:** Not applicable; infusing into oil requires more time than tincturing into alcohol. See Level 2: Infusing.
Level 2: Tincturing	**Level 2: Infusing**
Time: 1–3 days **Plant Type:** Thick and/or waxy leaves, such as citrus, bay, labdanum, rosemary, and conifers. These leaves need more time in the solvent than flowers do, but they still contain water (unless they're dried). As with flowers, wilt them slightly, under the same conditions.	**Time:** Cold: 1–3 weeks; Hot: 1 hour or less **Plant Type:** Fragile flowers, such as jasmine, violets, and roses. Thin leaves, such as mint, scented geraniums, and dried herbs. As with tincturing, wilt the botanicals slightly for up to an hour before infusing.
Level 3: Tincturing	**Level 3: Infusing**
Time: 1–2 weeks **Plant Type:** Hard, dense, woody materials, such as ambrette seeds, orrisroot, vetiver root, and clove buds. These materials need the most time in the solvent because the oils are encased in dry, tough, resistant botanicals.	**Time:** Cold: up to 8 weeks; Hot: a few hours **Plant Type:** Thick and/or waxy leaves included in Level 2 under tincturing and hard, dense, woody materials included in Level 3 under tincturing.

For plants that are not mentioned in this book, find a plant with a similar texture listed in Chapter 6, and use the steeping time for that plant, adjusting it as necessary.

STRENGTHENING YOUR TINCTURES AND INFUSIONS BY RECHARGING

The typical goal of tincturing and infusing is to make the most concentrated, highly-scented extrait possible. This requires recharging the solvent to increase the scent strength. Recharging means straining the botanical from the solvent and replacing it with more botanicals. To reach the highly-scented goal, you need to recharge your tincture or infusion at least several—possibly many—times before the solvent is properly scented. However, there are exceptions. Some botanicals will readily release enough scent with fewer recharges; these are noted in the individual plant briefs in Chapter 6.

You can also let your nose be your guide, especially when you're extracting scents from plants that are not mentioned in this book. The process for producing a highly-scented, all-natural perfume product is easy enough, and the rewards are great.

Most often, you will recharge your tincture or infusion until it is saturated, meaning that the solvent will not absorb any more scent. However, if you decide that the scent is strong enough, you may choose to stop the process before saturation. You'll learn this through experience.

STORING YOUR EXTRACTS

The requirements for storing most extracts are fairly simple. Keep them in a cool, dark place. I use a metal cabinet for most of mine, but you can store them anyplace (such as in a cupboard or on shelves), as long as they aren't in direct sunlight and are away from any heat source. However, some extracts require cooler storage, and it's best to refrigerate them.

Because of their high alcohol content, tinctures protected from light and heat can last for years. Refrigerate tinctures made from delicate flowers and herbs—such as lilacs, hyacinths, lily of the valley, rosemary, and lemon balm—so that they last longer. Because of their rarity and beauty, these tinctures are worth the shelf space in your refrigerator. Do this with any other tinctures that you feel are delicate.

Oil-based infusions aren't as shelf stable as alcohol-based extractions. Because of this, it's important to store your infusions even more carefully than you store tinctures, especially keeping them away from heat and sunlight. With careful storage, they will last a few years.

I've never refrigerated an infused oil, but if you're working with a more delicate one, or if you're reinfusing into an oil with a shorter shelf life, you can experiment with refrigerating your product.

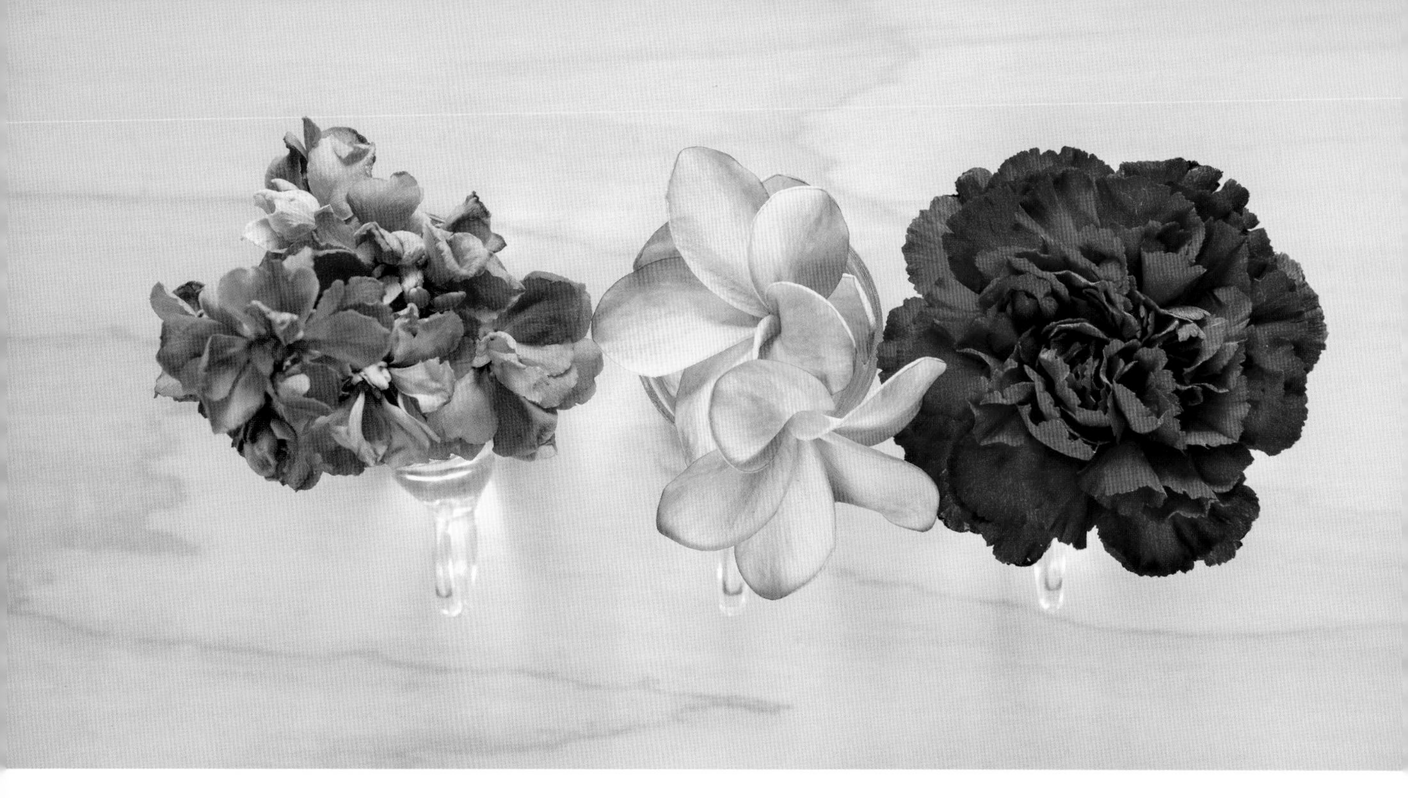

Claude Monet famously said, "I must have flowers, always, and always." I'll add that they must be fragrant! Some are so mysterious, they only reveal their scent at night, such as the night-scented stock shown above, so be prepared for nighttime harvests. Daytime beauties abound, though, so you have a wide time frame to pick the flowers. Shown from left to right: night-scented stock, plumeria (frangipani), and carnation.

MY TINCTURE OR INFUSION IS FINISHED: NOW WHAT?

You can use the alcohol tinctures as subtle substitutes for essential oils in perfume. Sometimes, if they're strong enough, they can completely substitute for essential oils, although their volume is greater, of course. You can take the tinctures one step further by using either the low-tech or high-tech extraction processes (see page 39). They can also be used in room, linen, and body sprays (see Chapter 5 for instructions).

You can use your infusion as a body oil as soon as you're finished creating it. If the scent is strong enough, you can use it as a base for oil or solid perfumes, for body butters, and in bath milk. A small amount rubbed between your palms and smoothed over your hair makes a scented hair conditioner and provides some shine. You can also blend your infusions together to create custom scents that please you. Let your creativity take over—the possibilities are endless!

TRADITIONAL VINEGAR EXTRACT

Vinegars selected for your projects can vary according to your personal preference. Apple cider vinegar is very popular, and if you make your own vinegar, all the better. Organic vinegars are easy to find or make, and if you have organic botanicals, you can make 100 percent organic scented vinegar. Note: Do not use distilled white vinegar. In the 1970s, I created my first facial vinegar made from apple cider vinegar and rose petals. It was so easy to make that I went on to experiment with different herbs and flowers for the scent and healing properties. I've used calendula petals, rosemary, mints, elderflowers, and even lemon slices.

MATERIALS AND EQUIPMENT

Fresh rose petals, rosemary sprigs, calendula flowers, mint, or the botanical of your choice, enough to pack the jar

Quart (950-ml) jar with a nonmetallic lid

Wooden spoon, chopstick, or metal skewer

Vinegar of your choice (except distilled white vinegar)

Labels and record-keeping tools

Scent strips

Stainless steel strainer

Filter papers (optional)

Decorative bottles with nonmetallic caps or corks, or plain jars

PROCESS

1. Pack the botanical in the jar very tightly, then push it down with the handle of a wooden spoon, a chopstick, or a metal skewer to compact it. Fill the remainder of the jar with the botanical to about 2 inches (5 cm) below the top of the jar.
2. Pour the vinegar in, pushing with the spoon again to release any air bubbles. Put the lid on and turn the jar upside down to release air bubbles. Don't skip this step because air pockets are susceptible to mold. Turn the jar right side up.
3. Make sure that the botanicals remain covered by the vinegar because any part of the plant that is exposed above it can grow mold. Label the jar with the plant names (both common and botanical), the date, and any other pertinent information, such as the extraction method, plant parts used (flowers, leaves, seeds, and so on), and the type of vinegar (such as apple cider, rice, or coconut).
4. Put the vinegar in a dark cabinet to age for four to six weeks. Check weekly to make sure the vinegar is still covering the botanical because some may be absorbed into the botanical, or evaporate. Top off with more vinegar if necessary. When you do the weekly check, gently shake or swirl the jar to expose the surface area of the botanical to the vinegar. Use the handle of a wooden spoon, chopstick, or skewer to break up any air bubbles.
5. After the required time needed for what plant materials you're using (refer to Level Methods Timetable chart on page 32), or when the plant material is spent, strain it—using filter paper placed inside the strainer if you choose—into either plain jars or decorative bottles. To test for scent strength, dip a scent strip into the vinegar. Either smell the vinegar on the scent strip, or dab some from the strip onto your hand and evaluate the scent on your skin.
6. If desired, recharge the vinegar with fresh plant material and repeat the steeping process once or twice. Because vinegar extracts are desired more for their healing properties, a strong scent from many recharges may not be necessary.
7. When you decide the vinegar is ready, label the container with all of the information from the first label, as well as the number of charges. Keep herbal vinegars in a dark cabinet because exposure to light causes them to lose their initial color. They will last for one to two years.

TRADITIONAL LOW-TECH ALCOHOL TINCTURE

This tincturing process is the oldest method of tincturing. It's also the simplest, requiring the least amount of equipment. For this method, your solvent is high-proof alcohol. See both the Levels Method Timetable (page 32) and the plant page in Chapter 6 for the specific botanical that you're tincturing to determine how long to steep it. If your plant isn't listed, choose a fragrant plant from Chapter 6 that is similar. Also, before you begin your tincture, make sure to properly prepare your botanical (see page 27).

MATERIALS AND EQUIPMENT

Botanical material

Wide-mouth jar with a tight-fitting lid

Wooden spoon, chopstick, or metal skewer

Alcohol (190 proof recommended)

Labels and record-keeping tools

Cheesecloth

Stainless steel strainer

Glass or stainless steel funnel

Scent strips

Filter papers

Sterile bottle or jar, for storing.

PROCESS

1. Place the prepared botanical into a jar, filling it about halfway. Lightly pack the botanical down by tamping it with the handle of a wooden spoon, a chopstick, or a metal skewer.
2. Add alcohol to at least 1 inch (2.5 cm) higher than the botanical, and tightly close the lid.
3. Label the jar with the plant names (both common and botanical), the date, and any other pertinent information, such as the extraction method, plant parts used (flowers, leaves, seeds, and so on), and the type of alcohol (if you use different types, such as grain, sugar, etc.).
4. Place the jar in a cool, dark place. Gently shake or swirl the jar at least twice daily to bathe the botanicals in the alcohol so that all of their surface areas come in contact with the alcohol.
5. When the plant material is spent, strain it from the alcohol through a piece of cheesecloth lining the strainer.
6. Using the funnel, pour the alcohol back into the jar. Recharge the alcohol with more plant material, and repeat the steeping process until the scent of the extract is to your liking. To test for scent strength, dip a scent strip into the alcohol. Either smell the tincture on the scent strip, or dab some from the strip onto your hand and evaluate the scent on your skin. Each time you recharge the solvent, make a note of it, both on the jar's label and in your notes.
7. When the tincture is finished, pre-wet a filter paper with 190-proof alcohol and place it into the strainer or funnel. (Pre-wetting the filter helps lessen the amount of scented alcohol being absorbed by the filter.) Filter the tincture into a sterilized bottle or jar. Label the container with all of the information from the first label, as well as the number of charges. Store the tincture in a cool, dark place. See "Storing Your Extracts" on page 33 for more plant- and solvent-specific storage details. You can use your tincture as is, or concentrate the scent further (see page 39).

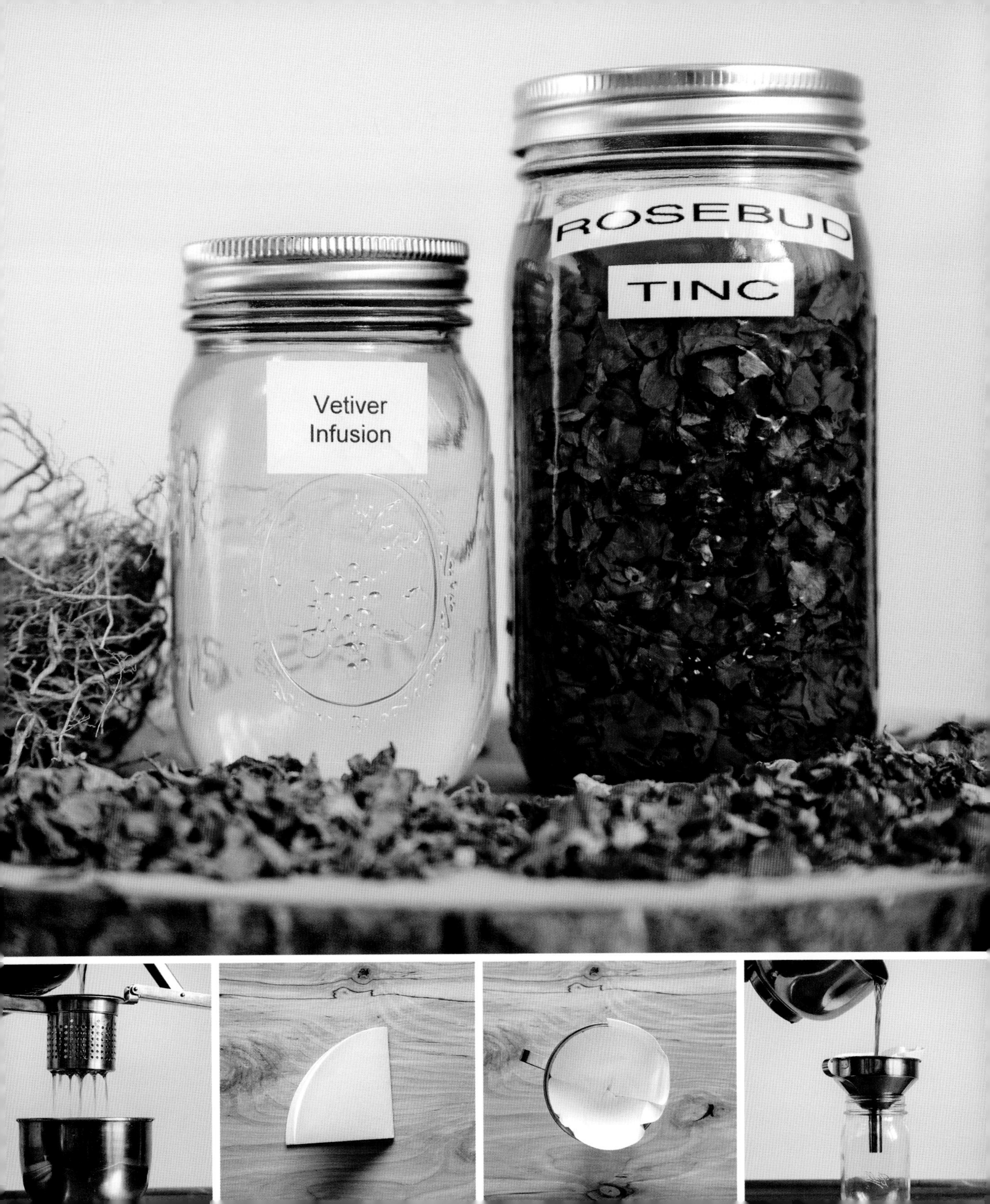
Vetiver
Infusion
ROSEBUD
TINC

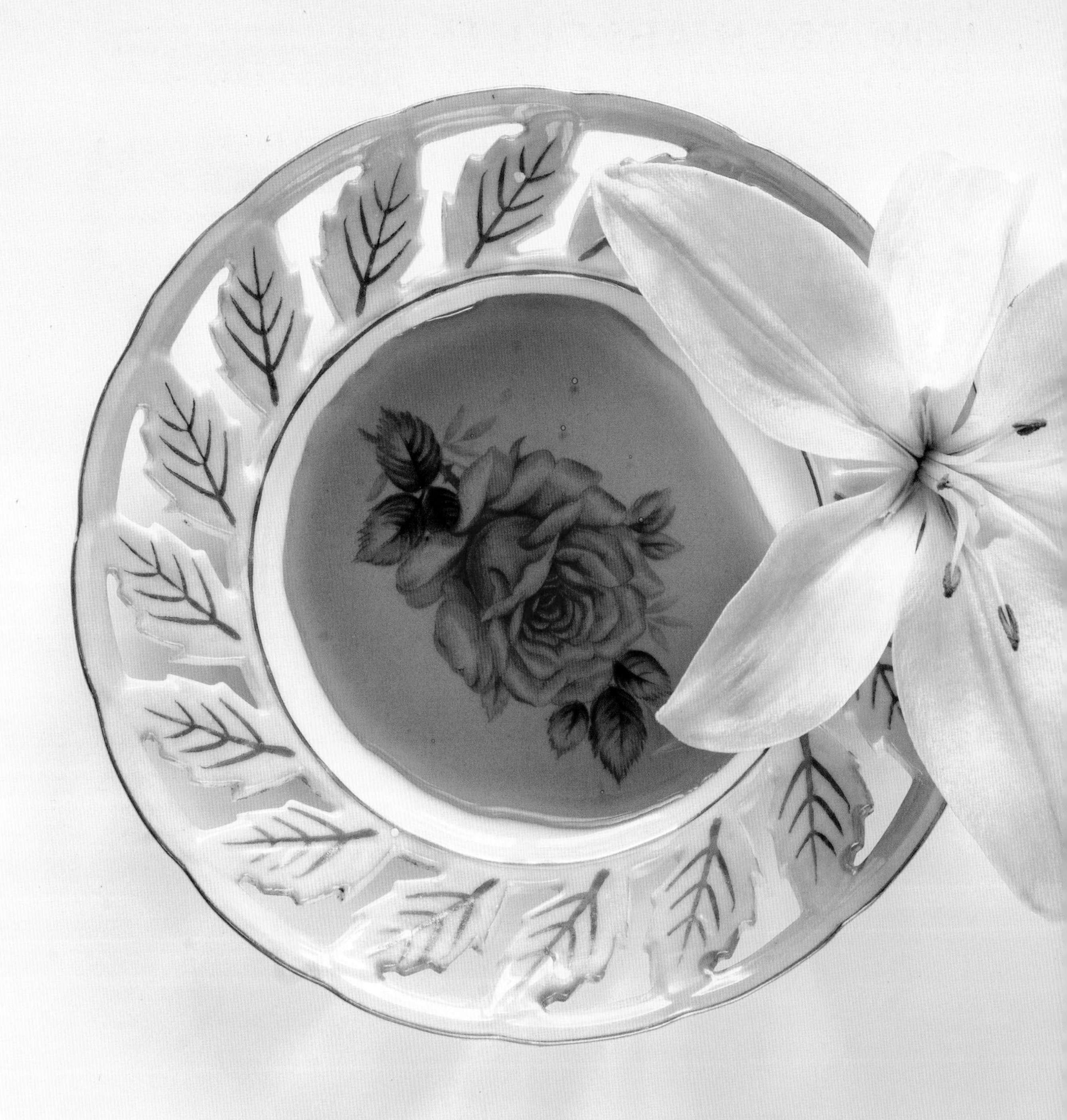

LOW-TECH ABSOLUTE OIL EXTRACTION FROM A TINCTURE

This is a method that I have used for years to evaporate the alcohol from a tincture, resulting in something very similar to an absolute oil. The procedure may not be feasible when the humidity is high, so try to conduct this evaporation process on a low-humidity day. Experiment first, using only a small amount of your tincture so that you don't lose all of your extrait if there is an accident, or if you make a mistake while you're learning how to do this in your own climate. Note: Because of the nature of this process, you will likely lose some of the top notes during evaporation.

MATERIALS AND EQUIPMENT

Scented tincture

Nonreactive deep plate or wide-mouth shallow jar

Cheesecloth or muslin

Labels and record-keeping tools

Left: Low-tech absolute oil extraction can be as simple as pouring your tincture (or clarified extrait from enfleurage) into a wide plate, dish, or jar and allowing the alcohol to evaporate off under controlled conditions. Not shown is the cloth cover to protect the liquid from dust while it is being processed.

PROCESS

1. Pour the tincture into a nonreactive, deep plate or a shallow jar.

TIP: If you decide to use a shallow jar, it's a good idea to use a canning jar with only the ring lid, which you can screw over a cheesecloth to keep small bugs out of the extrait.

2. Suspend or drape a porous cover over the plate or jar. I use a cheesecloth, muslin, or another breathable cloth. If possible, tuck the cheesecloth underneath the plate or jar to keep it secure. This step is unnecessary if you use a canning jar with cheesecloth.
3. Place the plate or jar on a flat surface, in an outdoor place that is protected from rain, and away from flame, or where it might be knocked over.
4. Check the extrait after one day; it may be ready. It should be reduced in volume and look thick and syrupy.
5. Label the container with the name and type of extrait and the date that it was made. Store it in a cool, dark place. See "Storing Your Extracts" on page 33 for more plant- and solvent-specific storage details.

HIGH-TECH ABSOLUTE OIL EXTRACTION FROM A TINCTURE

If you have a distillation system with a vacuum column, merely place the tincture into the distillation unit and distill the alcohol from the tincture, leaving behind the absolute oil. See "Vacuum Distillation" on page 53 and "High-Tech Absolute Oil Extraction—Vacuum Distillation" on page 87. When the extrait is finished, label the container with the name and type of extrait, and the date that it was made.

TRADITIONAL COLD OIL INFUSION

Cold oil infusion is the oldest and simplest method of infusing, requiring the least equipment. If you're very busy or, like me, a bit forgetful when it comes to paying attention to time, this no-worry technique is for you!

For this method, you use oil as your solvent. No measuring is necessary; just estimate the proper amount of plant material that will come to within an inch or two of the top of the jar and cover it with the solvent. To determine how long to steep the plant that you're infusing, see both the Levels Method Timetable (page 32) and the correct plant page in Chapter 6. If your plant isn't listed, choose one that is similar.

MATERIALS AND EQUIPMENT

- Botanical material
- Wide-mouth jar with a tight-fitting lid
- Wooden spoon handle, chopstick, or metal skewer
- Oil, such as moringa, argan, coconut, jojoba, or light olive
- Labels and record-keeping tools
- Stainless steel strainer
- Cheesecloth (optional) or coffee filter
- Glass or stainless steel funnel
- Nonreactive sterile bowl
- Scent strips
- Filter papers (optional)
- Sterile bottle or jar, for storing

PROCESS

1. Place the botanical into a jar, filling it about halfway. Lightly pack the botanical down by gently tamping it with the handle of a wooden spoon, a chopstick, or a metal skewer.
2. Pour the oil into the jar, covering the botanical, until the oil level is at least 1 inch (2.5 cm) higher than the botanical.
3. Tamp the botanical again and pour in more oil to cover the botanical by 1 inch (2.5 cm), making sure to remove any air bubbles from the plant and the oil—oxygen from air bubbles promotes microbial growth. Screw the lid on tightly.
4. Label the jar with the plant names (both common and botanical), the date, and any other pertinent information, such as the extraction method (cold oil infusion), plant parts used (flowers, leaves, seeds, and so on), and the type of oil (such as moringa).
5. Do not shake the infusion because it will create air bubbles. Every day or so, gently push the botanicals down in the oil with the sterilized handle of a wooden spoon, or other sterile implement, dispersing any visible air bubbles. See "Caution with Fresh Botanicals in Infusions" on page 29.
6. Watch to see when the flowers or leaves become limp and spent, or turn translucent (dried materials lose some color when spent, and may also get soft or softer to the touch). When this happens, strain them from the oil by pouring them into either a strainer lined with cheesecloth, or a funnel, allowing the scented oil to drain into a sterile bowl.
7. Return the oil to the jar. Recharge the oil with more plant material, and repeat the steeping process.

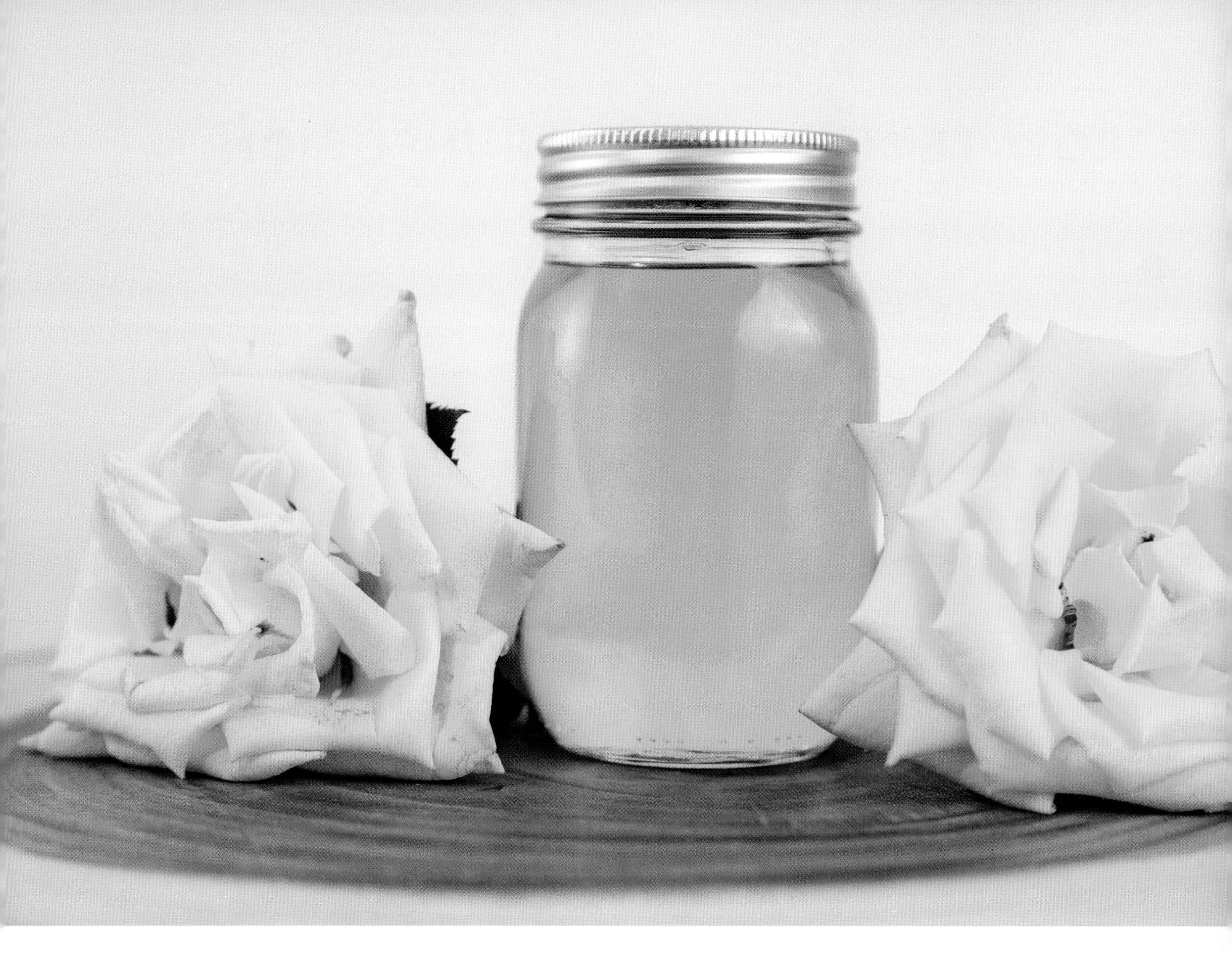

Rose scent is easy to extract in a cold oil infusion and makes a luxurious, beautiful oil for use alone, in an oil perfume, solid perfume, massage oil, hair oil, or body butter.

8. Continue recharging, steeping, and straining until the scent of the extract is to your liking. Each time you recharge the solvent, make a note of it, both on the jar's label and in your notes.
9. To test for scent strength, dip a scent strip into the oil. Either smell the oil on the scent strip, or dab some oil from the strip onto your hand and evaluate the scent on your skin. Note: Never put your fingers directly into the oil because this introduces contaminants.
10. When the infusion is finished, filter it, using filter paper if desired to ensure you capture every bit of botanical, then decant into a sterilized bottle or jar. Label the container with all of the information from the first label, as well as the number of charges. Store your infusion in a cool, dark place. See "Storing Your Extracts" on page 33 for more plant- and solvent-specific storage details.

LOW-TECH HOT SOLAR INFUSION

This solar infusion harnesses the heat of the sun to extract the scent from plants. It takes a few weeks, but it's so carefree that I think you'll love it.

MATERIALS AND EQUIPMENT

Botanical material

Jar with a tight-fitting lid

Wooden spoon, chopstick, or metal skewer

Oil, such as moringa, argan, coconut, jojoba, or light olive

Labels and record-keeping tools

Sterile jars

Pipette (optional)

Cheesecloth or coffee filter

Stainless steel strainer

Scent strips

Filter papers (optional)

PROCESS

1. Place the botanical into a jar, filling it about three-quarters of the way.
2. Lightly pack the botanical down by gently tamping it with the handle of a wooden spoon, a chopstick, or a metal skewer.
3. Pour the oil into the jar, covering the botanical until the oil level is at least 1 inch (2.5 cm) higher than the botanical.
4. Tamp the botanical again, making sure to remove any air bubbles from the plant and the oil (again, oxygen from air bubbles promotes microbial growth), and screw the lid on tightly.
5. Label the jar with the plant names (both common and botanical) and any other pertinent information, such as the plant parts used, type of oil, extraction method, and date.
6. Place the jar in a sunny spot on a windowsill or outside in an area where it is protected from rain, such as under an awning, but still able to receive several hours of sunlight a day. If you're using fresh plant material rather than dried botanicals, check the infusion daily for a water separation layer on the bottom of the jar. If that layer develops, carefully decant the top layer of oil and the plant material, and place it in a sterile jar. If there is some oil and water left in the jar, discard it or use the oil immediately.
7. You may also use a long pipette to pull the water from the bottom of the jar. (Make sure you get it all.) Do this daily until you don't see a water layer on the bottom. Most plant material will solar infuse in two weeks. Dried materials lose some color when spent, and may also get soft or softer to the touch.
8. Strain the plant material out using cheesecloth and a strainer, and recharge the oil as many times as needed until the desired scent strength is reached. Each time you recharge the solvent, keep a record of it in your notes. To test for scent strength, dip a scent strip into the oil. Either smell the oil on the scent strip, or dab some oil from the strip onto your hand and evaluate the scent on your skin.

NOTE: Never put your fingers directly into the oil because this introduces contaminants.

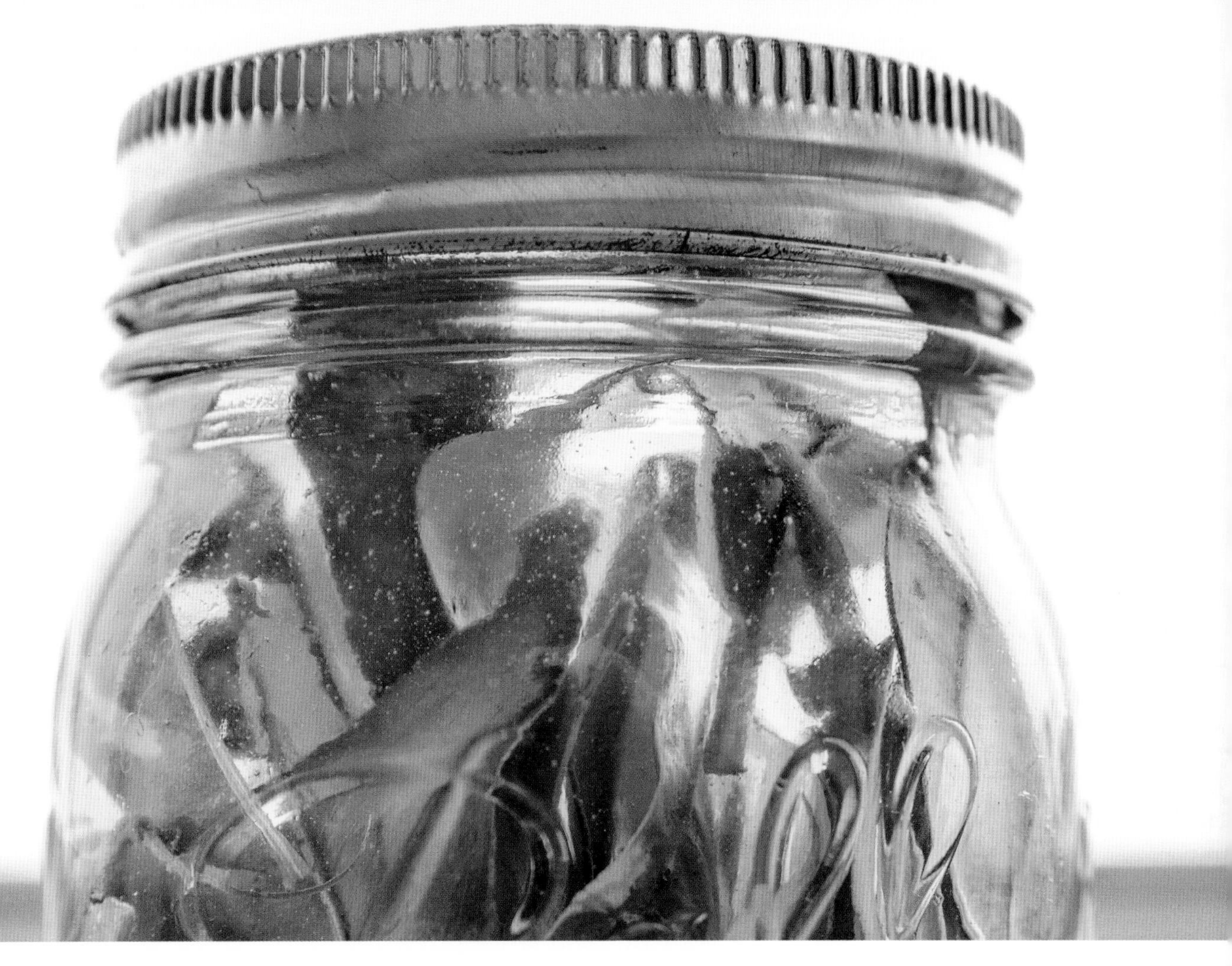

One of the easiest and historically oldest ways to extract scent from botanicals is solar infusion. Simply put your botanical in a jar, cover with oil, place a cap on it, and let it sit in a sunny window or outdoors in the sun where it is protected by an overhead awning or other covering. Shown here is a solar infusion with variegated lemon leaves.

9. After you achieve the desired scent strength, strain the final plant material using a strainer or cheesecloth, lined with filter paper for a clearer product, if you wish. Pour the oil into a sterile jar with a tight-fitting lid.
10. Label the jar with all of the information from the first label, as well as the number of charges, and store it in a cool, dark place until you're ready to use it. See "Storing Your Extracts" on page 33 for more plant- and solvent-specific storage details.

DOUBLE BOILER HOT INFUSION

Did you know that the double boiler method, also known as bain-marie, was first devised in ancient Egypt by a renowned herbalist and distiller named Maria? The French made this method popular in the kitchen for delicate dishes, such as custards, so "bain" in French means bath, and "Marie" is the French version of her name. She used this method to gently heat herbs and spices. Some herbs and spices are too delicate to take direct heat, or you may want to speed up the extraction time by devising a bain-marie.

Extracting plant material in a double boiler requires that you pay attention to the pot and not leave it unattended for more than a few minutes. Double boilers are easy to find and inexpensive. However, if you don't have one, it's easy to create a suitable makeshift version with two nonreactive pots. The top pot must have a tight-fitting lid.

MATERIALS AND EQUIPMENT

Botanical material

Oil, such as moringa, argan, coconut, jojoba, or light olive

Double boiler with a lid

Stainless steel strainer

Sterile jar or bowl

Scent strips

Glass or stainless steel funnel

Coffee filter or cheesecloth (optional)

Labels and record-keeping tools

PROCESS

1. Place the botanical and oil into the top pot of the double boiler and cover with a tight-fitting lid. Be sure that the oil completely covers the botanical. Fill the bottom pot with enough water to boil, but don't let it reach the bottom of the top pot. Place the top pot onto the bottom pot, and put the two onto a stove burner or hot plate. Place the lid on the top pot.
2. Bring the water to a low simmer, keeping the heat below 104°F (40°C). Periodically check the temperature of the oil and make certain that it remains below 104°F (40°C). If you have trouble maintaining this low oil temperature with your burner, there are inexpensive gas burner diffusion pads; I find them very handy for keeping the temperature low.
3. Process the plant material for several hours, periodically stirring it and checking the temperature. Make sure that the plant material is constantly covered by the oil so that no parts are exposed to air. Also, occasionally check the water level in the bottom pot.
4. When you see that the flowers or leaves are limp and spent, or have turned translucent, take the top pot off the heat and let the oil cool. Dried materials may become lighter in color and softer or limp in structure when spent.
5. Pour the oil and botanical into a stainless steel strainer and allow to drain into a jar or bowl.
6. Determine whether the oil needs recharging with fresh plant material to increase the scent strength. To test for scent strength, dip a scent strip into the oil. Either smell the oil on the scent strip, or dab some oil from the strip onto your hand and evaluate the scent on your skin. Note: Never put your fingers directly into the oil because this introduces contaminants.

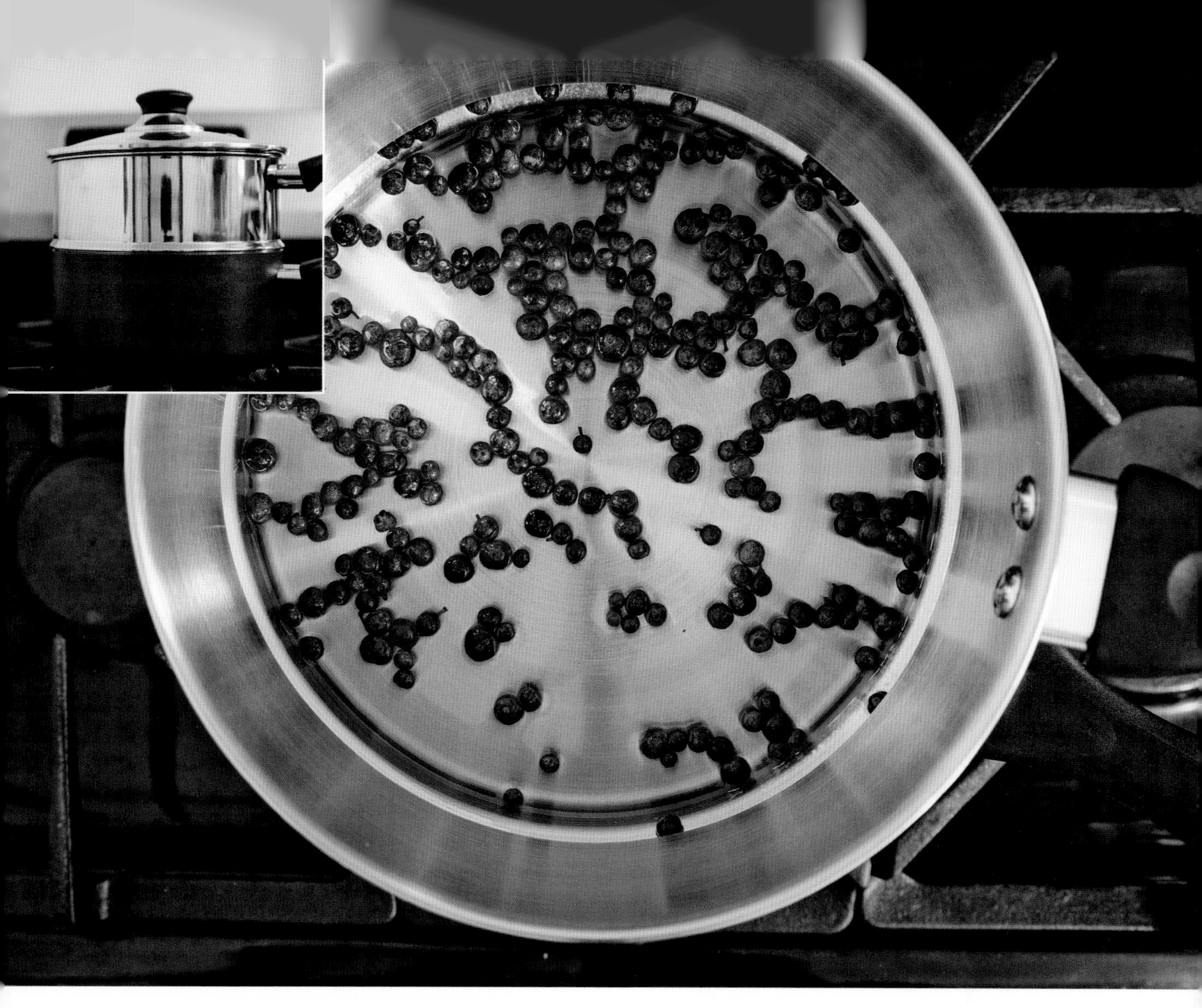

While some leaves and flowers are easy to solar or cold infuse, others—like hard seeds, woods, and roots—need additional heat to coax out the fragrance. Shown here are allspice seeds.

7. Strain and recharge the oil as many times as needed until the desired scent strength is reached. Each time you recharge the solvent, keep a record of it in your notes.
8. After the desired strength is reached, strain the plant material a final time, using a funnel and filter or cheesecloth, if necessary, to catch smaller pieces of plant material.
9. Pour the oil into a sterile jar with a tight-fitting lid. Label the jar with all of the pertinent information, such as plant names (common and botanical), parts used, type of oil used, extraction method, number of charges, and the date. Store the infused oil in a cool, dark place. See "Storing Your Extracts" on page 33 for more plant- and solvent-specific storage details.

SLOW COOKER HOT INFUSION

Using a slow cooker works well for hot infusions, but only if the heat of the slow cooker doesn't exceed 104°F (40°C). Note that because slow cookers can run too hot—even on the lowest setting—I typically use one only when I'm "hot" infusing a particularly tough raw material such as chopped dried vetiver roots or dried allspice berries. Even with tough botanicals, I run the slow cooker for only a short period, checking it frequently. This is where a heat-diffusing pad can come in handy. Place it in the slow cooker, and then place the bowl with the oil and botanical on top of the pad. Don't be afraid—let your passion and curiosity lead you to experiment like the many people who tinctured and infused in previous generations.

MATERIALS AND EQUIPMENT

Botanical material

Oil, such as moringa, argan, coconut, jojoba, or light olive

Heat-resistant bowl

Heat-diffusing pad

Slow cooker

Thermometer

Scent strips

Glass or stainless steel funnel

Stainless steel strainer

Clean jar or bowl

Cheesecloth (optional)

Sterile jar

Labels and record-keeping tools

PROCESS

1. Place the botanical and oil into a heat-resistant bowl, and place a heat-diffusing pad under that bowl in the slow cooker. The pad will create a space between the bowl and the slow cooker's pot, helping to keep the temperature low. Be sure that the oil completely covers the botanical.
2. Turn on the slow cooker to its lowest setting. Periodically check the temperature of the oil and make certain that it remains below 104°F (40°C). If you notice the temperature climbs too high, turn off the heat for a while to cool, then turn it back on. Process the botanical for several hours, stirring occasionally.
3. When you see that the botanicals are spent, or are not seeming to give off any more scent, remove the interior bowl containing the botanical from the exterior pot, and set it aside to cool. Dried materials may become lighter in color and softer or limp in structure when spent.
4. Determine whether the oil needs recharging with fresh plant material to increase the scent strength. To test for scent strength, dip a scent strip into the oil. Either smell the oil on the scent strip, or dab some oil from the strip onto your hand and evaluate the scent on your skin. Note: Never put your fingers directly into the oil because this introduces contaminants.
5. Using a funnel or strainer and a clean jar or bowl to receive the scented oil, strain and recharge the oil as many times as needed until the desired scent strength is reached. Each time you recharge the oil, keep a record of it in your notes.
6. After the desired strength is reached, strain the plant material a final time with a funnel or strainer, using a cheesecloth, if necessary, to catch smaller pieces of plant material.
7. Pour the oil into a sterile jar with a tight-fitting lid. Label the jar with the plant names (common and botanical), part(s) used (leaves, flowers, twigs, and so on), type of oil, extraction method, number of charges, and the date. Store the infused oil in a cool, dark place. See "Storing Your Extracts" on page 33 for more plant- and solvent-specific storage details.

DOUBLE BOILER AND SLOW COOKER COMBO HOT INFUSION

For most botanicals that aren't hard or woody, you can use a double boiler technique in a slow cooker. Simply place a smaller bowl containing the oil and plant material inside the slow cooker's ceramic pot that contains water. This is a trick that allows you to control a very low temperature a little more easily than either method alone. You may need to stand the smaller bowl on a metal rack in the slow cooker to raise it from the bottom of the larger pot.

MATERIALS AND EQUIPMENT

Botanical material

Oil, such as moringa, argan, coconut, jojoba, or light olive

Small bowl with a lid

Slow cooker

Thermometer

Metal rack

Scent strips

Glass or stainless steel funnel

Stainless steel strainer

Clean jar or bowl

Cheesecloth (optional)

Sterile jar with a lid

Labels and record-keeping tools

PROCESS

1. Place the botanical and oil into the small bowl and cover it with a tight-fitting lid. Be sure that the oil completely covers the botanical.
2. Place the pot into the slow cooker and fill the slow cooker with water one-third of the way up the side of the bowl.
3. Turn on the slow cooker to its lowest setting. Periodically check the temperature of the oil and make certain that it remains below 104°F (40°C). Be careful whenever you remove the lid that no water drips into the oil.
4. When you see that the botanicals are spent, or are not seeming to give off any more scent, remove the interior bowl from the slow cooker and set it aside to cool on a metal rack. Because of the variable nature of this method, you need to use your judgment for each infusion's finish time.
5. Determine whether the oil needs recharging with fresh plant material to increase the scent strength. To test for scent strength, dip a scent strip into the oil. Either smell the oil on the scent strip, or dab some oil from the strip onto your hand and evaluate the scent on your skin. Note: Never put your fingers directly into the oil because this introduces contaminants.
6. Using a funnel or strainer and a clean jar or bowl to receive the scented oil, strain and recharge the oil as many times as needed until the desired scent strength is reached. Each time you recharge the oil, keep a record of it in your notes.
7. After the desired strength is reached, strain the plant material a final time, using a cheesecloth, if necessary, to catch smaller pieces of plant material.
8. Pour the oil into a sterile jar with a tight-fitting lid. Label the jar with all of the pertinent information, such as plant names (common and botanical), parts used, type of oil used, extraction method, number of charges, and the date. Store the infused oil in a cool, dark place. See "Storing Your Extracts" on page 33 for more plant- and solvent-specific storage details.

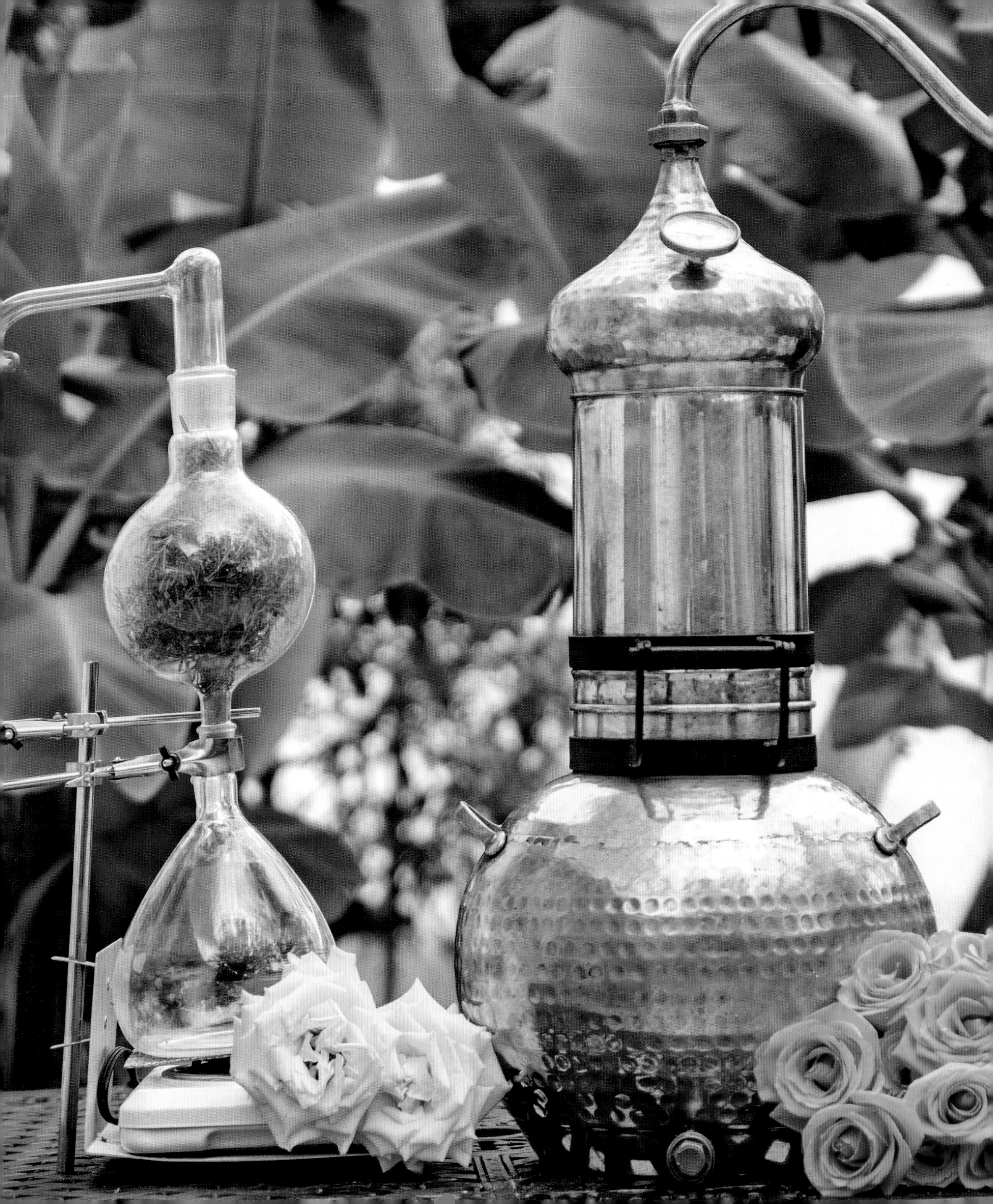

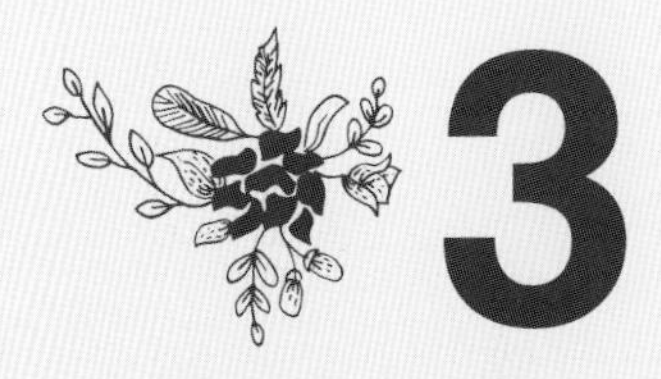

3

DISTILLATION

Essential oils are very popular today, but did you know their production and use are thousands of years old? It's wonderful to see the upsurge in interest in this method, and the careful use and enjoyment of these concentrated oils. Perfumers use these oils every day, but they are often purchased from suppliers because the amount of plant material needed is huge, and the yield often tiny. When making your own, you'll obtain a small amount of essential oil, and a larger amount of scented hydrosol, the water that comes along in the process. This chapter provides a good introduction to this fascinating art.

A fun fact is that, aside from plant material, various other substances can be distilled, such as seashells, soil (yes, dirt!), leather, and pretty much anything that can be put into a still.

Left: There are many sizes and types of stills available. I have two that serve my purposes, and I encourage you to read more, contact suppliers, and decide which is best for you. Shown here from left to right are a 2-liter glass steam still (with rosemary in the steam chamber) and a 20-liter copper steam-and-hydro still.

INTRODUCTION TO DISTILLATION

Distillation is the most complex extraction method in this book, requiring a fair amount of expertise, or a willingness to tackle a steep learning curve. The methods of distillation for the different types of extraction and the variety of stills that are currently available warrant an entire book to themselves. But don't be discouraged when I mention steep learning curve and expertise: I include a fast, low-cost, no-still method of creating scented hydrosols on your stove top or electric hot plate (see page 59). You won't get any essential oil, but hydrosols are great for many fragrant uses. I make this "simplers'" hydrosol at least once a week—it's addictive!

To distill a botanical, the plant is either combined with water in a distillation unit or suspended above water. When heat is applied to the distillation unit, the water temperature rises, creating steam and releasing the aromatic molecules from the botanical. The scent molecules are carried along with the steam through a chilled condenser that causes the vapor to revert to liquid. This liquid is the volatile scented oil of the plant and the water that holds water-soluble molecules. The liquid flows either into a receiving vessel, where the oil floats on top of the water and is siphoned off, or into a separatory vessel that has two different outlets—one for the essential oil and one for the hydrosol water.

A still is an extraction system made of several pieces of equipment connected in series, which, when used in perfumery, processes extraction material, usually with water and/or steam, to produce scented extracts. From their earliest crude clay distillation alembics, distillers experimented, and their distillation units evolved to use different materials, such as copper, steel, and glass. Modern units may have a gauge to monitor the temperature, vacuum columns for specialty distillations, and a separatory flask to easily separate essential oil from water distillate.

INTRODUCTION TO ESSENTIAL OILS AND HYDROSOLS

Distillation produces two products: an essential oil and a hydrosol. Some distillers adjust their stills to produce more essential oils; others may prefer to produce only a hydrosol.

Essential Oil

Also called volatile oil or ethereal oil, essential oil is the fragrant plant essence that gives each plant its characteristic scent. When you smell a mint leaf, or a rose, or the rind of an orange, you're smelling the essential oil. Depending on the plant, essential oils are obtained from various parts (flowers, leaves, roots, or bark) by steam or hydro-distillation, the two primary distillation methods that you'll learn more about soon.

The typical yield of essential oil from plant material is 1 to 3 percent by weight. Even though most people don't have access to the kilograms of rose petals that are needed to distill a single ounce (30 ml) of rose oil, this book presents an option that can produce a few drops of rose oil. If you distill volatile, oil-rich dried products—such as vetiver root—you may get a few milliliters, so don't give up on the idea of distillation because of the lack of a large still and lots of plants.

Hydrosol

When plant material is steam or water distilled, a portion of the extracted scent and natural constituents that include scent molecules remain in the distillate water, which is called hydrosol. The hydrosol has scent and taste properties and is useful for many perfumery projects, including body and face sprays, room and linen sprays, and colognes.

For centuries, distilling rose petals and orange flowers resulted in the only two hydrosols that were sold to the consumer: rose water and orange flower water. Currently, a variety of these waters are sold to consumers, and they are used in aromatherapy, cosmetics, and food. The scent molecules in hydrosols represent the less concentrated, more finely dispersed components of the plant material, and their fragrance is often beautiful, just fainter and less concentrated than that of the essential oils.

In the past ten years or so, artisan natural perfumers and distillers decided to try something new. They distill whatever they wish: fragrant fruit, cocoa nibs, gardenias, violets, and other nontraditional items. While many of these botanicals are too delicate to produce an essential oil by distillation, they're producing a hydrosol for the pleasure of having a scented water that's useful in health and beauty products.

Although these hydrosols may be much less potent than an essential oil, they uniquely showcase materials that do not yield essential oils. The elusive fragrances of various fruits, flowers, roots, and seeds are now flowing from artisan stills around the world, lending new and unusual beauty to the world of aromatics.

Traditional and Modern Uses for Hydrosols

Hydrosols can be used on their own as room, linen, or body sprays. They can be sprayed on the entire body, including the hair, providing a subtle, overall perfume, and can be added to a perfume or cologne, where their fragrance will contribute gentle nuances to the blend.

Hydrosol is a combination product, often embodying aspects of the essential oil, but also containing many healing, water-soluble compounds that are not present in the essential oil. This makes hydrosols popular in the world of body care and cosmetics.

You may wish to keep a spray bottle of a hydrosol in the refrigerator to spray on your face for a refreshing spritz. Because hydrosols have a relatively short shelf life, they are not meant to be stored for—or used over—a long period of time. Refrigeration is always recommended.

Popular Hydrosols

The following botanicals are most often distilled for hydrosol. I encourage you to experiment with distilling other botanicals for hydrosol.

- Basil
- Bay laurel
- Calendula
- Frankincense
- Jasmine
- Lavender
- Lemon balm
- Lemon verbena
- Mint
- Myrrh
- Orange (or other citrus) blossom
- Rose
- Rose geranium
- Rosemary
- Sandalwood

Safety with Hydrosols

Exercise the utmost caution in keeping all distillation glassware sterile if you don't plan to use preservatives in your hydrosols. These delicate beauties are easily contaminated and need careful handling from still to bottle. See "Safely Cleaning Equipment for Projects" on page 21.

Hydrosols must be produced and maintained in sterile conditions, especially if they're used for body care or food and beverage additions. This means that the following precautions must be observed:

1. Quickly recap the jar or bottle after opening to lessen the introduction of airborne particles or microbes.
2. Do not put your fingers into the hydrosol bottle.
3. Be mindful of keeping the hydrosol as sterile as possible.
4. Do not store hydrosols for more than two weeks, even with refrigeration.

Some distillers monitor the pH of their hydrosols. If the initial pH begins to rise and become more alkaline, it indicates that the hydrosol is beginning to "turn" or "bloom" with microbial growth. You may wish to have your hydrosols tested for microbial activity. See Appendix 3 for recommendations.

If you use hydrosols in your perfumed products, you might consider adding a preservative—such as alcohol—to them to prevent spoilage. You can research further on your own to decide whether to use them in this manner.

METHODS OF DISTILLATION

As the practice of scent distillation evolved, so did different methods of distillation. To better extract fragrance for each type of product, several methods of distillation are used, dictated by the type of plant (or other) material. Let's unpack each of them.

Hydro-Distillation

This is the oldest distillation method, and it is most useful for distilling tougher herbs, woods, roots, seeds, and powdered spices, as well as some flowers, such as roses, which are exclusively hydro-distilled. The plant material is added to water in a retort or boiling cylinder. The botanical material must be able to withstand the heat and pressure of boiling.

Small distillers often use this method because of its simplicity and reduced cost. However, hydro-distillation can be tricky because it is difficult to maintain a consistent distillation rate. Material near the bottom of the still can be overheated, giving the product a burned note. Additionally, hydrolysis—a chemical reaction with the water—can occur, which ruins delicate, fruity-smelling plant compounds. Some botanicals are never hydro-distilled because they lose their sweet, fruity aspects in the process.

Steam Distillation

For this method, also called water/steam distillation, the aromatic plants are placed in a separate vessel above the one containing the water. Steam from the water vessel passes through the botanical in the vessel above it and is collected in the condenser. In a simple steam distillation setup, the botanical material is separated from the steam-producing hot water by a fine mesh grid. You can steam distill just about anything, except for roses because they clump into a mass and can scorch.

Vacuum Distillation

This method uses a special adapter, called a vacuum column, which is attached to the distillation unit. During distillation, the vacuum column reduces the atmospheric pressure above the distillation chamber, allowing extraction to occur at temperatures that are below the normal boiling point and often at room temperature. This is a desirable way to distill aromatics because there is no danger of scorching them.

Vacuum distillation is an important procedure in the creation of certain isolates. It is also used to remove the alcohol from tinctures, creating absolute oils, which are the highest-quality distilled extraits.

WHAT YOU NEED TO BEGIN DISTILLING

Before you can begin distilling, you will need a number of items, including the distillation unit or system and additional pieces of equipment, tools, and materials. You will also need to spend some time studying how to distill before you begin.

Unless you have a good understanding of distillation and are a bit mechanically inclined, the setup, actual distillation, and collection of the final product can be daunting. There are many books, YouTube videos, and websites that can help you understand the process, and numerous teachers conduct distillation workshops. Free publications on distillation are also available; just search the Internet or your local public library for them.

Distillation is the only process for which I specifically recommend that two people work together, at least until you become adept at distilling. Once you become comfortable with the process, distillation can be a wonderful solo project. Start small and work your way up, especially if you plan to distill for essential oil.

Distillation Units/Stills

Distillation units are now easily available from the Internet and in shops in some locales. The size and type of unit you choose are dictated mainly by your budget and the type of product you wish to make. You will need to research the best distillation method for your particular plant material before obtaining the appropriate unit. A small stove top still may suffice for the modern apartment dweller who wants to experiment with this ancient art by producing hydrosols. You need a much larger unit to obtain essential oil because the yield of most botanicals is extremely low, sometimes less than 1 percent of the biomass of the botanical. This could mean that after completely filling the bioflask of a small tabletop still unit, the end result from a distillation is only two to three drops of essential oil.

If you are a bit mechanical and you like the idea of creating a distillation system, you can make one from old coffeemaker carafes, saucepans, or pressure cookers, with the help of some instructions from YouTube videos. I don't have the nerve for this, but I encourage you to experiment and try some different methods if you are so inclined.

You can find still-making instructions online. One method is to adapt a pressure cooker. However, if you use this method, you must be sure to know what you are doing. There are very real dangers if your system is built or assembled incorrectly because you are working with pressure and steam.

I have two distillation devices: a 2-liter glass steam distillation unit and a 20-liter copper hydro- or steam distillation unit. Sometimes it is a bit of a bother to set them up, so when I just want to make a quick hydrosol, I don't set up my distillation units. Instead, I use a method that was probably used thousands of years ago and remains efficient and productive today. I call it the Simplers' Hydrosol Distillation method, and you need only a few basic kitchen tools. It's a terrific project for a beginner who's interested in trying out distillation but not ready to buy a still yet. You'll find the step-by-step instructions on page 59, but make sure to read through the rest of this introduction first so you know what other tools you'll need and how to properly prepare certain botanicals for distilling.

Additional Equipment, Tools, and Materials

Aside from the distillation unit itself, you'll need some additional equipment, including the following:

Glass bottles: You should have bottles on hand in a variety of sizes for capturing the distillate. You can estimate how many jars or bottles you will need based on the size of the still and the amount of water that you add for either steam or hydro-distillation. It is best to collect distillates in a narrow-mouthed container rather than a canning jar. The narrower the opening, the less likely airborne bacteria and fungus spores are to drop into the container. Store in clear bottles; this way you can easily look into the jar to see whether strands or spores of mold, clumps of fungus, or pathogens have accumulated. Sterilize the container by using a UV disinfection unit, such as those used by tattoo artists and aestheticians, boiling the container, or cleaning it with bleach. (See "Safely Cleaning Equipment for Projects" on page 21.)

Ice bath: This is required to cool the condenser coil. The ice bath consists of a large bucket or container filled with ice and water. Alternatively, you can use cold running water.

Separatory funnel: This is used to separate essential oil from hydrosol. A Florentine separator is also good for larger-scale distillation because it allows the hydrosol to keep flowing while oil accumulates.

Pipettes: These are used to separate essential oil from hydrosol.

Sealant: This is necessary for sealing joints between still parts against any air leaks. A good homemade option is rye flour. When mixed with water, the mixture creates a putty that provides a quick seal for alembic still leaks. Rye flour is best because putties made with other flours tend to crack under the heat of the distillation. Modern distillers use silicone tape for sealing still joints.

Cleaners: Distillation units require cleaning to remove residue between projects. White vinegar cleans well as long as there is no resinous residue. You can also use grain alcohol. Simply dilute 1 cup (237 ml) of alcohol with 1 gallon (3.8 L) of water. Distill this through the unit to dissolve residue from inside the still parts.

Tubing: This is used to transport water to and from the condenser from the ice bath.

Submersible pump: This is necessary to pump water in the tubing.

PREPARING BOTANICALS FOR DISTILLATION

The quality and yield of your end products are directly affected by the care with which you treat the botanicals. Before putting them into the still, you need to prepare them properly. See specific plant briefs in Chapter 6 for information on what time of day to harvest (if applicable). Fresh botanicals are typically used in distillation, but some materials, including roses, benefit from slight wilting.

Even distribution and tight packing are necessary for steam to pass evenly through the mass of plant material. Without this consideration, steam cuts preferential channels through the charge and much of the plant material remains untouched by the steam. Distill your plant matter directly after preparing it to avoid excessive loss of essential oil to evaporation from newly exposed surface areas.

Here are a few tips for distilling certain types of plants:

- Herbs give a better yield if they're chopped before distillation.
- Flowers that are tiny or fragile, such as roses or elderflowers, should be distilled immediately after harvest.
- Woods, roots, and dried spices release their essential oils better if they're soaked in water before distillation. They also benefit from chopping and grinding.
- Conifer needles may need soaking in hot water for several hours, or partial drying prior to extraction, to break up the waxy cuticle that protects the essential oil glands.
- Fruits, such as mangoes and cantaloupes, should be cut into small pieces for distillation. Again, this is a new trend, so have fun and experiment.

DISTILLATION TIMES

The time needed to run the still can vary greatly, depending on the plant material, the desired end result, and the size of the distillation unit. During any distillation process, pay attention to the smells emanating from your distillation unit. Learn to smell what distillers call the head, middle, and tail of the scent. The best scent is typically found in the head or middle. The tail of the scent is often flat and may smell overcooked.

The head scent appears shortly after the steam starts and is typically very pleasant and smells like the plant. The middle is perhaps a bit deeper, still pleasant, and signals that the distillation is about to go into the tail phase. You want to stop the process as soon as you detect the tail, or right before that moment if you can. The goal is head and middle distillates, which will give you the highest-quality scent.

Older distillation books recommend using high heat and high pressure. However, distilling is not a one-size-fits-all process. High heat and high pressure could produce a great yield, or it could easily scorch the botanical. The new generation of artisan distillers is obtaining beautiful results by carefully monitoring temperatures, listening to the still, smelling what's coming from the still, and using their judgment. I see more distillers of herbs and flowers moving toward low temperature and low pressure for a slow and easy still run. High temperature and pressure is the typical distillation method for essential oils, while low and slow is more typical for hydrosols. The current theory is that many aromatics that are water soluble are slower to distill.

This chapter presents two very basic distillation processes to get you started (see pages 59 and 60). There is much more to learn, and I encourage you to research thoroughly in order to get the biggest and highest-quality yield from the system you have. I research each time I distill a new botanical, and there's always something to learn. I highly recommend joining some artisan distillation Facebook groups, where members share experiences and you can ask specific questions, post photos of your setup, and get to know others in the distillation community.

STORING YOUR ESSENTIAL OILS AND HYDROSOLS

As with the storage of infusions and tinctures, essential oils and hydrosols need a dark, cool place, like a cabinet. Make sure the lids are on tightly, and they will last for a long time. The only difference in storage will be if you have refrigerator space. Be aware that the scent from the essential oils will be a bit strong. For this reason, I have a separate refrigerator for storage. I didn't need one at the beginning, but as time went by and I had more and more goodies to preserve, I needed to move beyond my little spare cube refrigerator and buy a full-size unit for the garage. Be prepared: If the natural fragrance "bug" catches you, you'll eventually need one, too.

REMINDER: When you remove something from the fridge, allow it to come to room temperature before lifting the lid. Otherwise, condensation may form, and when you replace the lid, water will enter your product and may cause it to go bad.

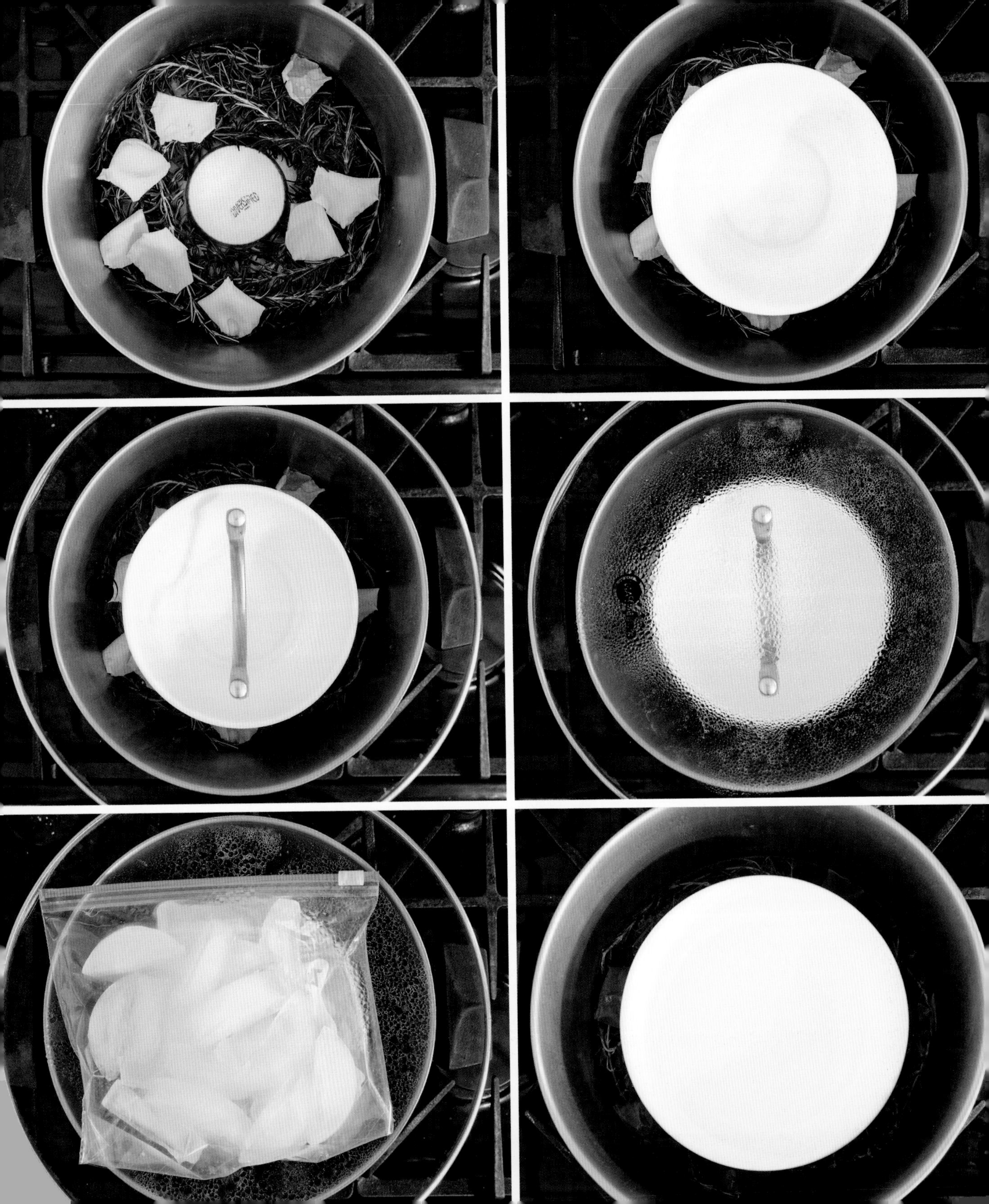

SIMPLERS' HYDROSOL DISTILLATION

Before you jump into buying a still, here's something you can do tonight with simple kitchen equipment, some ice, and, of course, some fresh botanicals. I use this process weekly, because of its ease of use and instant reward. I call it a simplers' distillation, paying homage to the simplers' method of herbal tincturing and infusion. That means nothing is measured; the botanical is simply covered with the solvent—water. This distillation process works with either a stove top, hot plate, or campfire. Note that all of the equipment must be made of nonreactive material, such as stainless steel, enamel, heat-resistant glass, or ceramic.

MATERIALS AND EQUIPMENT

Large pot or saucepan

Platform to elevate the bowl, such as a custard cup with a flat bottom

Plant material (fresh is best, but you can experiment with seeds, bark, roots, and other dried material)

Filtered water

Bowl that fits inside the pot or saucepan

Pot lid with a slight dome (cannot be flat) and glass or metal handle (not plastic)

Zip-lock plastic bag

Ice to fill the plastic bag (you may need to refill the bag several times as the ice melts, so have a generous supply available)

Sterile container for the finished hydrosol

Labels and record-keeping tools

PROCESS

1. Place the pot or saucepan on the stovetop, hot plate, or other heat source.
2. Center the elevation platform in the bottom of the pot. It's important that the platform be as small as possible because the area around it must be large enough to hold as much plant material as possible. I use an upside-down custard cup with a flat bottom.
3. Place the plant material around the platform, up to the top of the platform. Pack it gently to fit as much as possible in the space without damaging the botanical.
4. Add enough water to cover the plant material by 1 inch (2.5 cm).
5. Place the bowl on the platform. This is what will collect your hydrosol. Make sure there is at least 1 inch (2.5 cm) of space between the bowl and the sides of the pot, allowing steam to rise around it.
6. Put the inverted lid on the pot, with the dome facing downward, to allow the steam to drip into the bowl.
7. Bring the water to a boil over high heat, then lower the heat to medium.
8. Fill the zip-lock bag with ice and place it on the inverted lid. Make sure to use a zip-lock bag that's big enough to cover the lid but does not spill over the sides.
9. Maintain a strong simmer, hot enough to maintain the steam, but not a furious boil, which will damage or scorch the plant material. Replace the bag of ice as needed with fresh bags of ice.
10. The distillation is finished when the plant material looks "spent," or when your nose detects no more scent that you identify with the plant. Take the pot from the heat and remove the bag of ice from the lid. I put the bag back in the freezer for the next distillation.
11. Keep the lid on and allow the pot's contents to cool to room temperature. Pour the hydrosol from the bowl into a sterile container and close it tightly. Label the container with the date, plant material, and extraction method used. Store in a cool, dry place. See "Storing Your Essential Oils and Hydrosols" on page 57.

A BASIC DISTILLATION PROCESS

You've researched what kind of still is best for you, and now you're ready to learn distilling and produce some beautiful scented products. This project describes the most basic process for a general still run to give you a good idea of how to distill. It also lists all the equipment and materials that you might need.

However, these are merely general guidelines. There are so many types of stills, and so many permutations of distilling, depending on which end product you're distilling for—essential oil, hydrosol, or both together—as well as which products you will make with the extrait. Follow the manufacturer's instructions for your particular distillation unit.

MATERIALS AND EQUIPMENT

Botanical

Distillation unit

Filtered water and ice to fill condenser

Thermometer

Sterilized bottles or jars to collect hydrosol and essential oil and to store end products

Clean cloth

Clock

Pipettes (for drawing essential oil from the top of the hydrosol)

Labels and record-keeping tools

PROCESS

1. Start by placing the botanical in the proper receptacle whether it's for hydro- or steam distillation. In some stills, this will be in the bottom bowl (the retort), in others the steam column, and in some both. Follow your still's instructions to get it set up for correct and safe distillation.
2. Fill the retort with filtered water according to the still's instructions. If you have good-quality tap water available, you may use this, but make sure there is no chlorine and the pH of the water is not alkaline. Attach the input and output tubes that carry cold water in and hot water out through the condenser. Turn on the submersible pump in a cooler filled with ice.
3. Start with the lowest temperature possible, as long as it produces steam. If your unit does not have a built-in thermometer, you will have to estimate the temperature.
4. Gradually increase the heat and monitor how the fragrance changes as the distillation progresses.
5. Place a sterile bottle or jar to catch the distillate as it flows from the condenser spout. Also place a clean cloth over the condenser spout and top of the jar to prevent microbes and dust from entering the collection bottle or jar.
6. Check periodically to ensure the ice has not melted, and add more when needed.
7. Keep precise notes on each still run using a clock so that you know what works best for temperature and time.
8. When the distillation is over, allow the hydrosol and oil some time to separate, and using a sterile pipette, draw the essential oil off the top of the hydrosol and bottle separately. Store your hydrosols in properly labeled, sterile containers. See "Storing Your Essential Oils and Hydrosols" on page 57.

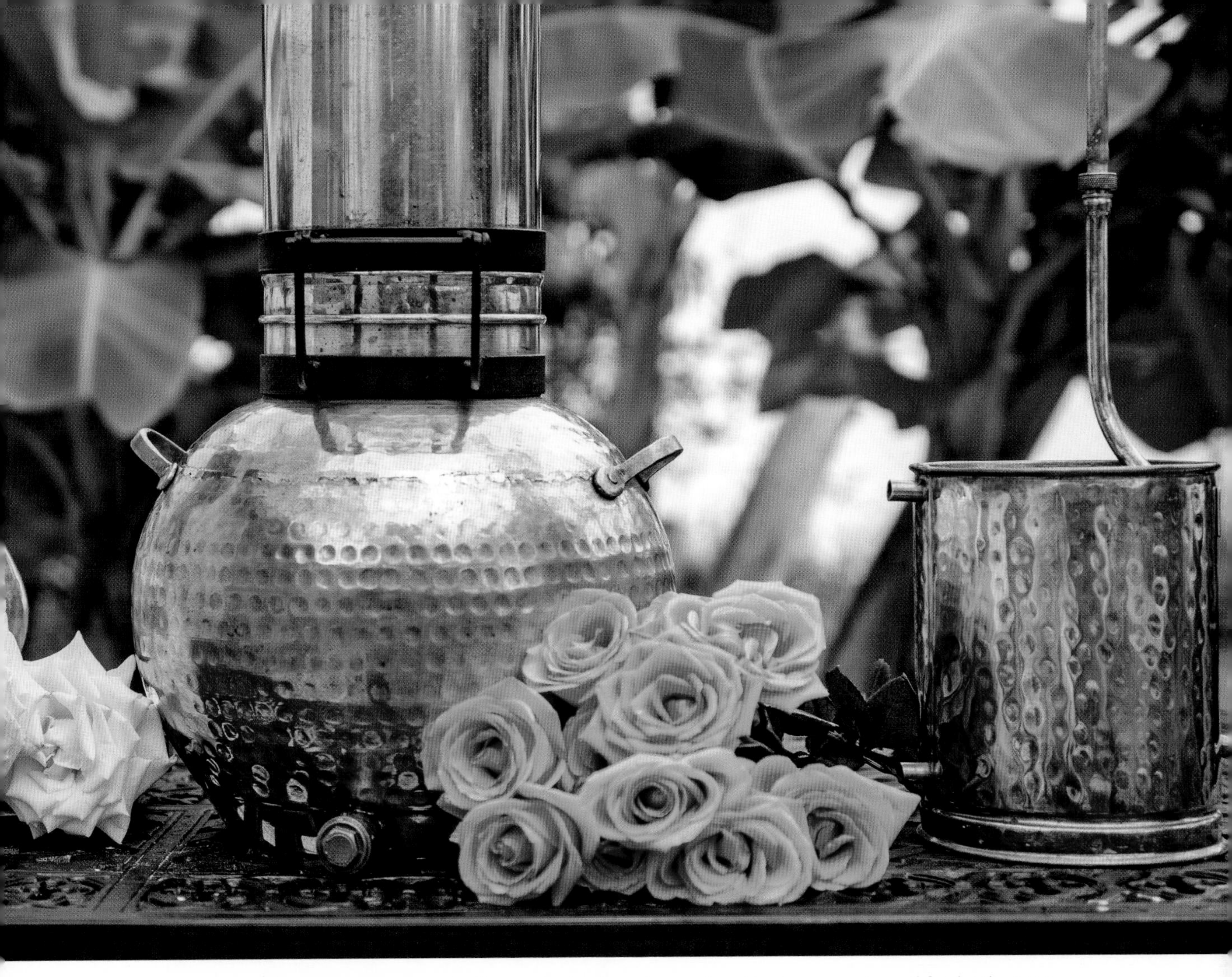

Copper stills can connect you to the ancient art and are often the type most used for both steam and hydro-distillation.

TIP: In any distillation, the condenser temperature matters just as much as the burner and steam temperatures. If the condenser water is too cold, the essential oils congeal and are difficult to separate from the hydrosol. The average temperature at which most oils readily separate from hydrosol is 110°F (43°C), give or take a degree. For example, with roses you must keep the condenser warm (not hot) so that certain aromatic compounds don't crystallize inside the condenser coils. You can learn a great deal while distilling a given plant by creating mental associations with specific odors and temperatures. Also keep in mind that the scent you detect during distillation will vary at different temperatures.

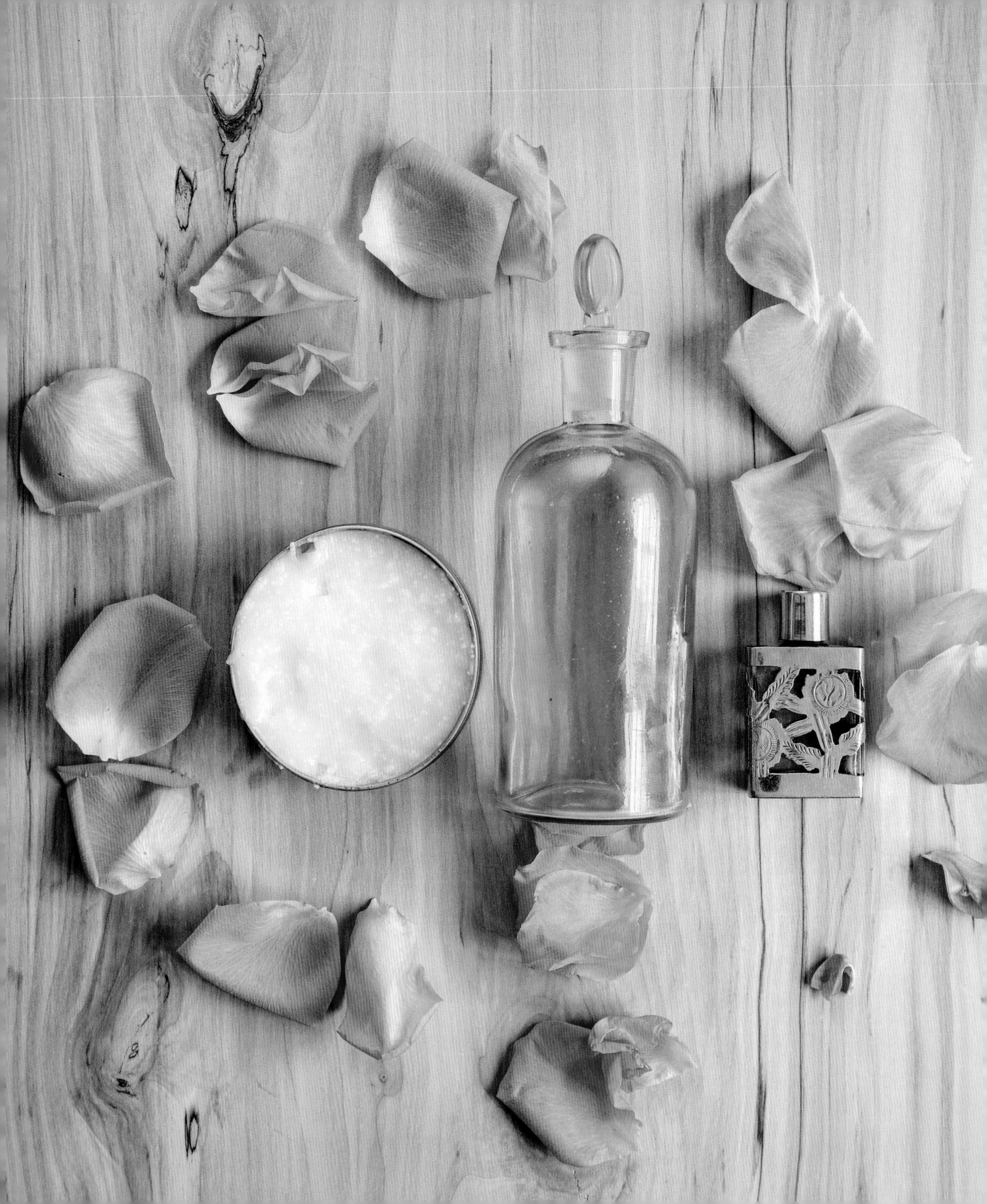

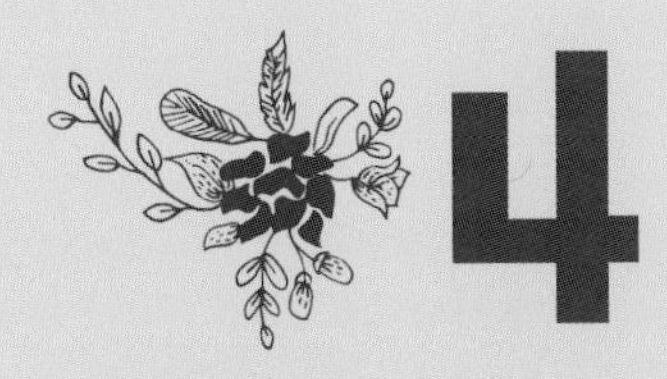

4

ENFLEURAGE

Enfleurage is such a gentle, rewarding way to extract the scent from fresh flowers. This method draws the scent molecules from a botanical into heated oil (maceration) or cool, room temperature semi-solid fat (pomade). I've also experimented with powder and resins, which I write about, but flowers in oil or semi-solid fat are true enfleurage. The oil or fat can be used "as is" for body oil, perfumes, or body butters, or processed further to extract the scent into alcohol.

For me, this method is so rewarding because it is the most effective way to obtain the true scent of the flowers, other than tincturing. Maceration (steeping plants in heated oil) can be seen as an adaptation of a basic oil infusion with flowers, but it is more effective, yielding a highly desirable product. Plus, it's also much quicker. The flowers' scent is often altered by other extraction methods, such as distillation, and a lot of the top notes are lost, but not so with enfleurage.

Left: Scented pomade is a glorious, unctuous natural fragrance product that you can use right out of the jar, or you can process it further by "washing" with alcohol to extract the extrait, a clear, highly-scented liquid alcohol. Want to make absolute oil, such as the one in the little silver perfume bottle? Further low- or high-tech extraction is needed. Shown here from left to right is scented pomade, a bottle containing alcohol extrait of pomade, and a perfume bottle with absolute oil after final processing.

INTRODUCTION TO ENFLEURAGE

There is currently a revival of the artisanal practice of enfleurage. It was abandoned by the commercial industry in the twentieth century upon the discovery of solvent extraction, which was more cost-effective. The beauty and art of enfleurage are both easy and sensually pleasing for the perfumer to accomplish. The act of picking the flowers (or buying them from a trusted supplier), preparing the enfleurage receptacle with the fat, placing the flowers onto—or into—the fat, and providing successive recharges is, to me, a soothing and contemplative process that also links me to perfumers of the past.

Small-scale enfleurage is quite inexpensive, and with the purchase of only a few easily obtained materials and items of equipment, you can begin extracting the scent from flowers. You'll need an airtight or nearly airtight container, the fat (and, if you're in a warm climate, a stiffening agent—often beeswax), and the flowers. The process of placing the flowers on the fat, allowing enough time for the scent to bond to the fat, removing the flowers, and replacing them with new ones (recharging the fat) might be repeated dozens of times to perfume the fat with a desired strength of scent. This book will give you ideas for more spontaneous and, perhaps, unconventional containers to use, and you may even devise a new type yourself.

The beauty of enfleurage is that you can choose how far to process it for your end products because each stage of the extraction process yields a product that is ready to use without any further processing, though you can certainly process the extraction further.

There are several end products that a fat or oil enfleurage yields:

- **Pomade:** A fragrant semi-solid fat that extracts the volatile oils from flowers. It is such a luscious product, sensual and usable just "as is." It can be used to make body butters and solid perfumes and soaps, or it can be an addition to solid perfumes or balms. Pomade can be further processed to extract the fragrant oil and "extrait."

- **Extrait:** Obtained by "washing" the pomade in alcohol. The washing may take several weeks of agitating the mixture to draw the scent out of the fat into the alcohol. The agitation can be as simple as shaking the jar several times a day, or using a mechanical device. The pomade extrait is a type of tincture that is made by tincturing the volatile oils from the fat or oil into the alcohol, and processing them further with vacuum distillation or simply allowing the alcohol to evaporate under controlled conditions.

- **Absolute oil:** Evaporated or vacuum distilled from the extrait. The distillation evaporates the alcohol, resulting in a pure absolute oil that is completely soluble in alcohol, suitable for fine perfumes, with no cloudiness when blended. It will not become cloudy in cold temperatures either.

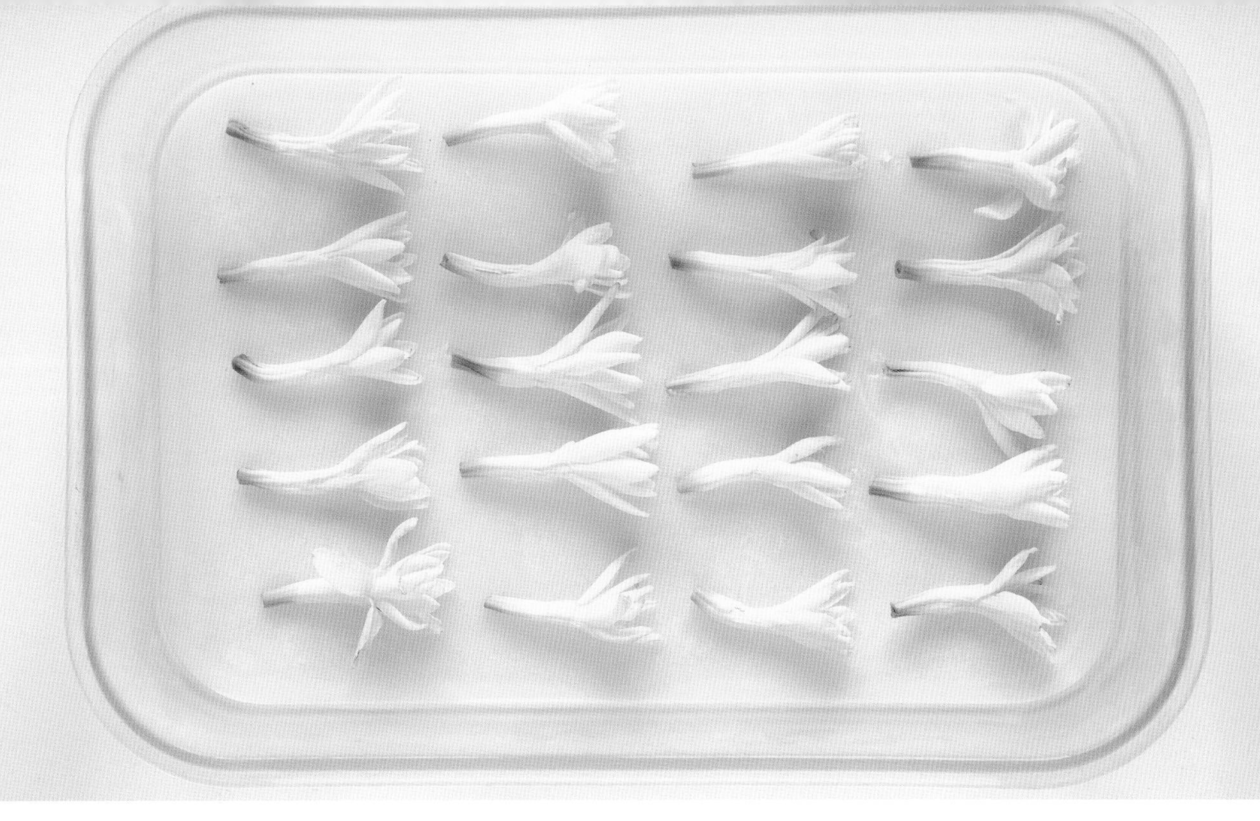

Flowers that "breathe" their fragrance over several days yield generously if enfleuraged. Tuberose (shown here) is a good example, as the flowers continue to exhale their fragrance for several days after picking. These beauties are placed on prepared pomade fat and then covered. In this picture, the tuberose flowers are on their second day and have become slightly opened.

TYPES OF ENFLEURAGE

There are several methods of enfleurage, using a variety of adsorbents for the flowers' scent molecules to adhere to. Enfleurage is conducted as either a cold or hot process. Some flowers work better with specific enfleurage methods. See Chapter 6 for method suggestions for each plant.

Cold Enfleurage Using Solid Fat

The cold processes for enfleurage that are covered in this book are fairly passive, low-labor activities for which you don't have to watch the extraction closely during the entire process. Cold enfleurage is conducted in four stages, without using heat.

With modern cold enfleurage methods, you typically place the flowers in the fat until they look translucent, or no longer give off scent. The time varies, according to the type of flower. As with infusing and tincturing, you can recharge the fat with fresh flowers once they become spent, allowing the fat to become saturated with scent. You can then use the pomade as is, or further process it to create an extrait, and eventually an absolute oil.

If you are using flowers that are too tiny or delicate to place directly on the fat, here's a tip. Place the flowers in a wire basket or fabric mesh bag, then suspend that in the large-volume container to hold the flowers near, but not in, the fat. This spares the garden perfumer the arduous task of removing many tiny flowers from the fat with tweezers.

If you have whole flowers that are too large to fit into a traditional enfleurage tray, what I call large-container enfleurage is a great solution. I first came across this idea when talking with a natural perfumer friend, Elise. She wanted to capture the scent of the peonies in her mother's garden. Because there weren't many blooms at the time, she didn't have enough for several recharges of a tincture, and there was no oil on hand for an infusion. Traditional enfleurage was out of the question because the large, full, round peony wouldn't fit into the enfleurage trays or plates that some artisans use. So, Elise grabbed a large plastic cup from her mother's cupboard, applied vegetable shortening to the cup's bottom and sides, inserted the peony, and put a lid on it. Voilà! A new and ingenious way—born of necessity—to achieve enfleurage in the world of the twenty-first-century natural perfumer! Elise and I have both used this technique with large flowers—like lilacs, roses, carnations, lilies, and gardenias—with terrific success, and I'm delighted to pass on the technique to you.

Enfleurage des Poudres

Scentless, smooth, and silky powders have been used for centuries as body powders. For the two decades I've spent in perfumery forums and discussion groups, read ancient perfumery books, followed blogs, and spoken with perfumers, nobody has written about, or mentioned, this ancient method of making them. Because many artisan perfumers around the world are reviving enfleurage, I am happy to share this most ancient enfleurage practice.

Powder enfleurage transfers the flowers' fragrance to powder, rather than fat, by adding fresh flowers to dry extraction materials, resulting in a beautifully scented product. Imagine capturing the scent of your summer roses, lavender, or other delicious plants in powder, then using the results as gifts.

TIP: Truly exciting is how lily of the valley flowers and lilac flowers, which can be a bit problematic when using pomade enfleurage, create a gorgeous powder product. Powder enfleurage is the quickest and simplest way to draw the fragrance of botanicals into a usable product—an excellent fragrant body powder, or dusting powder, like what our mothers and grandmothers used when we were little. With adult supervision, this extraction process is easy for small children to follow.

According to Dr. Y. R. Naves and G. Mazuyer in their wonderful book *Natural Perfume Materials*, plant powders in ancient times that were typically used included orris, ambrette, and oakmoss; starch and *faecula* (a starchy sediment extracted from food plants); and minerals such as talc. Common flowers used were jasmine, hyacinth, jonquil, orange flower, rose, mignonette, tuberose, lilac, wallflower, and lily of the valley. By a similar process, even hides and gloves were perfumed with the same flowers, as well as with violet and crimson carnation. It is to these long-abandoned methods that we trace the modern experiments with enfleurage. Talc is generally not used for this purpose anymore because asbestos is sometimes unavoidably intermingled with the talc during the mining process. Many people avoid cornstarch because most of the corn grown in the United States is genetically modified. There are several readily available alternatives that absorb moisture well. Tapioca starch (powder) and rice flour are commonly sold in Asian markets at reasonable prices, and arrowroot powder is known to have the silkiest "slip," thus feeling the smoothest on skin.

TIP: Mix the powder of a base note, such as orrisroot, into the tapioca starch or arrowroot. It really helps to capture the scent and extend the life of the scent.

Hot Enfleurage Using Warm Oil—or "Maceration"

Because the hot method of enfleurage that is covered in this book involves heating the fat and monitoring the temperature, it requires more active observation of the extraction process. However, the heat allows you to complete the process more quickly, which may be advantageous when you have a lot of flowers in bloom at once, or if the flowering period is short, such as with lilacs.

In French perfumery, maceration is the action of placing delicate flowers into warmed oil for a specified period of time. The flowers are strained out, and a new batch of flowers is placed in the oil. This recharging process is repeated several times, until the desired scent strength is reached.

TIP: Don't confuse hot enfleurage with hot infusions. While they are similar methods, hot infusion can be used to extract scent from flowers, as well as all other botanical materials such as leaves, roots, and resins, whereas hot enfleurage is for flowers only.

Vapor Essence Powder Enfleurage

Because I have a smoke allergy, I was delighted when natural incense maker and perfumer Katlyn, of Mermade Magickal Arts, introduced an incense and resin electrical warmer to the market. The device gently warms formed incense, loose incense, or resin chunks, releasing the scent of the aromatic in the manner that burning incense does, only without the smoke. I was finally able to have my home fragranced with blended incenses, as well as pure resins, such as frankincense, myrrh, copal, and opoponax. This device can be used to extract these scents into powder, without introducing the smoke scent that comes from burning incense.

NOTE: Even better, this warmer allows you to make scented powders from botanicals, such as the resins, which was impossible before.

MATERIALS AND EQUIPMENT NEEDED FOR ENFLEURAGE

This section presents all the necessary—and some optional—materials, equipment, and tools that you can use for enfleurage extraction.

Flowers: Most often, these are flowers that continue to "exhale" their scent after they're harvested. Traditional enfleurage flowers include jasmine, hyacinth, tuberose, mimosa, rose, frangipani, and gardenia. You may find a suitable flower in your garden by testing the fragrance and longevity of the blossom for a few days after it is picked. If the scent still wafts around a room after two or three days of being in a vase of water, it's a good candidate for enfleurage. Flowers must also have fairly sturdy, thick petals that won't wilt or decompose quickly. With the exception of rose, which can be distilled, the flowers I just named do not distill well because they cook, rather than release, their scent.

Fat: If the finished pomade will be used directly on the body, I suggest using only vegetable fats because friends, family, or customers may not wish to wear animal fat products on their skin. If, on the other hand, you plan to further process the pomade, it's fine to use animal fats.

Enfleurage vessel and covering: There are many items that you can use to contain the fat and flowers during enfleurage. The lids can be foil, glass, or plastic wrap. Pyrex plates with snap-on airtight lids are ideal. Here are several easy options for vessels:

- Stainless steel or glass (nonreactive) tray or a shallow pan with a 1-inch (2.5-cm) minimum depth
- Dinner plates
- Stacked-tray dehydrator unit, with all the vents sealed (use ceramic plates inside the unit to hold the fat and flowers)
- Trays from restaurant steam tables
- Glass jars of various sizes, ranging from small canning jars for powder enfleurage to ½- to 1-gallon (1.9- to 3.8-L) jars for large-container enfleurage

190-proof alcohol: This is necessary for washing the scent molecules from the pomade.

Tweezers: Use these for removing small flowers and bits of flowers and pollen from the corps, which is the fat of the pomade.

Airtight jars: These are necessary for processing and/or storing the pomade.

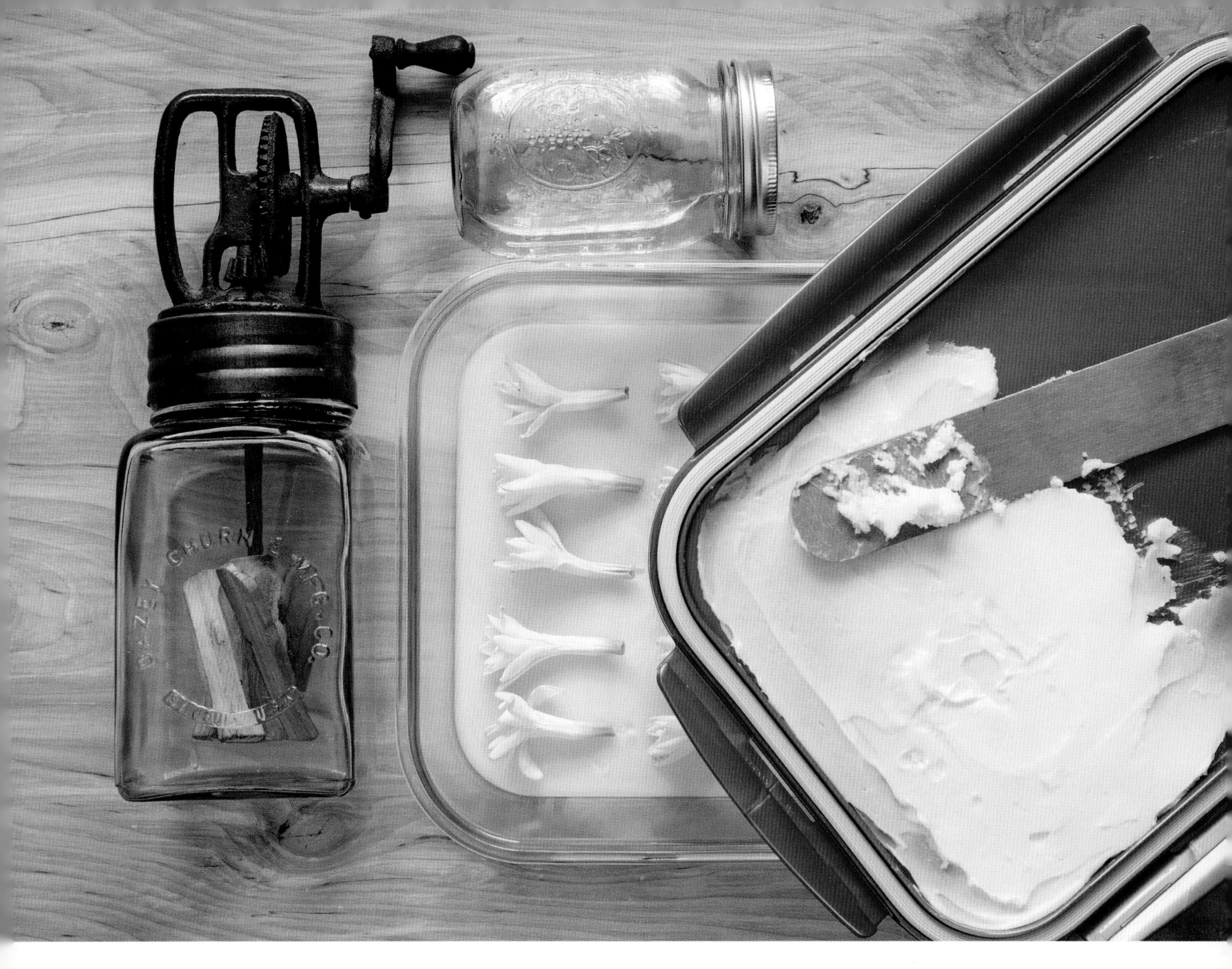

What fun when the DIYer finds an adaptive reuse for a common object! The mini butter churn shown on the left is for churning the finished pomade with alcohol. Since the tuberose flower is able to give up extra scent molecules, coat the inside of the lid using an offset spatula, as shown—a good use of all the container real estate.

Washing apparatus (optional): Agitation for washing the pomade can be accomplished mechanically by using a small butter churn (either hand- or electric-powered). Also, a non-planetary kitchen stand mixer can be modified to perform this task. A non-planetary mixer, in which the beaters are in a fixed position, lets you operate it with a lid on it. This cover reduces evaporation as much as possible. Many models are available with a stainless steel bowl and plastic snap-on lid for under $30. As long as you keep the alcohol and pomade mixture from splashing the plastic, it is relatively nonreactive. If you don't have access to a churn or mixer, simply shake the jar containing the pomade and alcohol mixture several times a day.

Labels and recordkeeping tools: As with all other perfumery projects, you'll want labels, a notebook, and a waterproof pen to record information for your reference later.

PREPARING FAT FOR COLD PROCESS ENFLEURAGE

In the art of enfleurage, the fat is known as the "corps" (core). For brevity, I refer to the solvent or adsorbent in this process as fat, regardless of whether it is a fat, an oil, or a butter. Traditionally, the corps was made from rendered beef or pork fat (suet and lard, respectively). The suet, pork "leaf fat" (from the kidneys), or regular lard was gently heated, sieved, then poured into enfleurage trays and allowed to reharden before the flowers were added. If you wish to use these products, I advise not to use them in body butters. Instead, wash the pomade with alcohol, and use the extrait.

Most modern-day perfumers use a semi-solid, scentless vegetable fat, such as deodorized coconut oil (kept below 75°F [24°C] so that it remains solid), non-hydrogenated vegetable shortening, or mango butter (which may be brittle to work with). However, you can use any of the vegetable fats that are available. If you wish, you can use scented fat, such as organic, unrefined coconut oil, but that will affect the scent of the flowers.

If you are in a cold climate, or you place the trays in a refrigerator to process, the consistency of the fat will support the weight of the flowers. However, if you are in a warmer climate, and your enfleurage container will be kept at room temperature, the bed of fat might be too soft, allowing the flowers to sink into it and making their removal difficult.

To obtain the proper firmness of fat for the enfleurage container in a warm climate, it's necessary to add a small amount of beeswax to the fat—this slightly hardens the fat. However, the beeswax must be used sparingly because it will trap scent molecules, and it's extremely difficult to separate the scent from the wax in the wash or distillation step. I highly recommend the granulated, or "bead," form of beeswax. It is so much easier to use and measure than the block form.

Steps for adding beeswax to fat:

1. Gently warm the fat until it melts.
2. Measure enough beeswax to equal 5 to 10 percent of the fat.
3. Add the beeswax to the melted fat, and stir until it dissolves.
4. Pour the fat into the enfleurage vessel and allow it to cool. You can refrigerate it to speed the cooling.
5. Optional: After the fat cools, score it in crisscross patterns, about 2 inches (5 cm) apart to a depth of ¼ inch (6 mm), using a tool such as a knife to increase the available surface area to which scent molecules can adhere.
6. Proceed with the flowers of your choice.

PREPARING FLOWERS FOR ENFLEURAGE

The quality of your end products is directly affected by the care with which you treat the flowers. Before putting them onto or into the fat or oil, you need to prepare them properly. See specific plant briefs in Chapter 6 for information on what time of day to harvest, if applicable. It's best to harvest the flowers when they are dry, rather than after a rain or when morning dew is on them.

Plants will need to be wilted before using them for enfleurage. This process is the same as wilting flowers for infusions and tinctures. The basic steps are to first harvest the flowers, taking care not to bruise them. Then, prepare a drying rack, an oven rack, or any flat surface by covering it with a cheesecloth or another porous material. Lay the flowers on the drying rack to wilt. If they are particularly moist (such as lush, dense flowers), this may take awhile. The flowers are ready for enfleurage when they look slightly softer and wilted, but not distressed or turning brown.

CAUTION: Do not wilt delicate flowers for more than an hour, or they can lose their most subtle top notes. Pay close attention to the scent, look, and feel of the botanical during wilting.

STRENGTHENING YOUR ENFLEURAGE

Traditional French enfleurage trays were often charged with fresh flowers 36 times. But not too many people nowadays have access to that many flowers, or the time and energy to recharge 36 times! Do what you can with what you have. The pomade can be stored under refrigeration until the next session of blooms, either from your garden or purchased. I recommend using a separate refrigerator for your perfume projects, as the scent can end up perfuming the food in your regular kitchen refrigerator.

You may wish to do fewer charges, so use your nose to determine when the pomade's scent reaches the appropriate strength. I have found that sometimes as few as six are needed to obtain a beautiful, usable product, but many of my pomades require at least a dozen.

STORING YOUR ENFLEURAGE POMADES AND EXTRAITS

Historically in France, pomades were stored in caves, where the temperature was cool and stable. To get the same effect for these delicate products today, I always store pomades and alcohol extraits in tightly sealed jars in a refrigerator. Whenever you need to remove a pomade or extrait from the refrigerator, allow the container to remain unopened for 24 hours so that the temperature equalizes with the room temperature in order to avoid condensation. Condensation produces water, which, if allowed to drip into the product, can cause mold. Using a disinfected or sterile implement, remove the amount of pomade you need, then immediately reseal the jar and return it to the refrigerator.

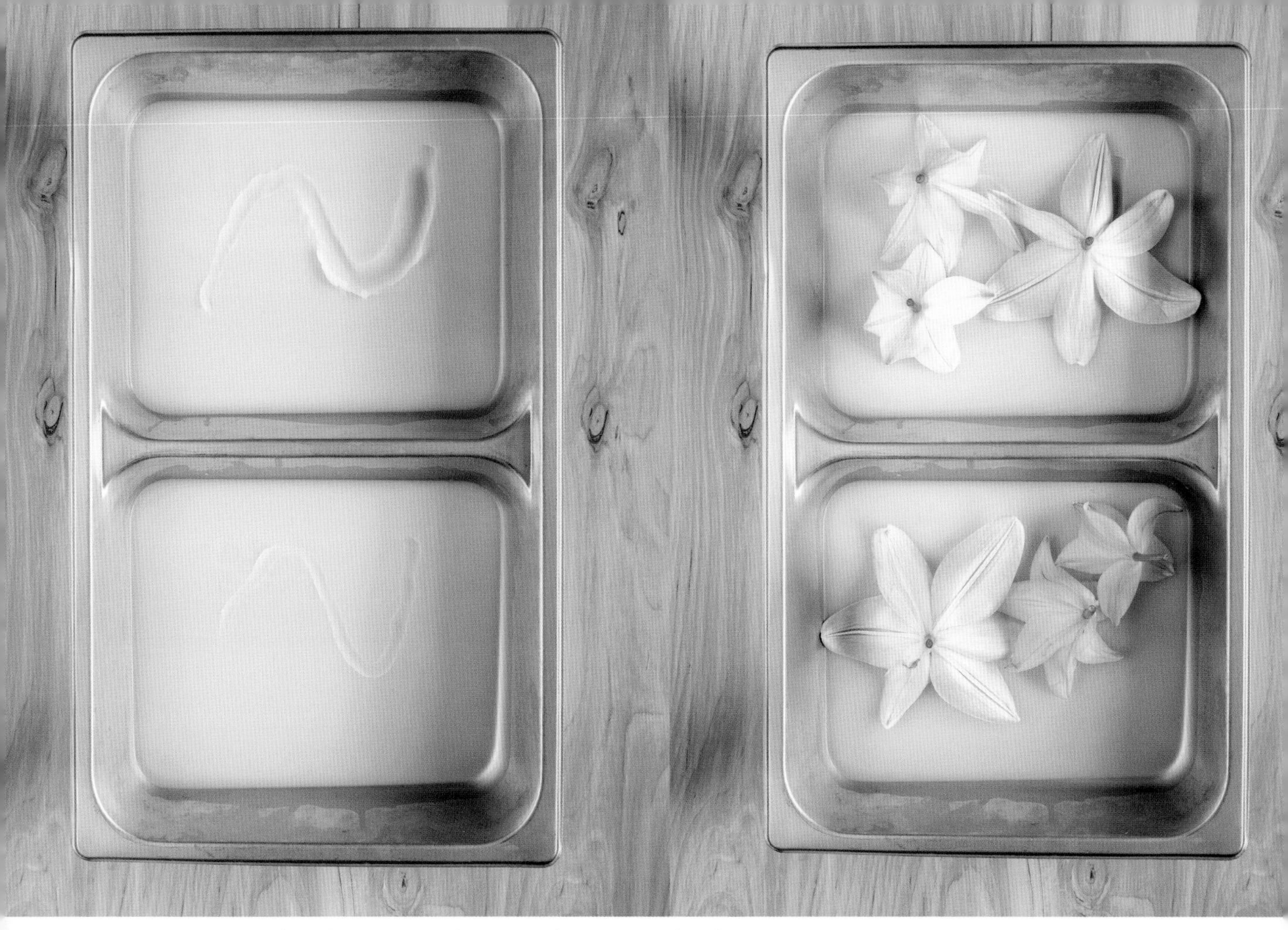

Here's a quick and easy way to figure out if your pomade is firm enough. The upper tray on the left shows too-soft pomade. I lightly drew my finger through it, which left a deep impression. The bottom half has enough beeswax melted into the fat to provide a firmer texture. Look how much shallower the impression is. On the right are two properly-prepared, firm pomades with lovely lilies sitting on it for scent extraction.

TRADITIONAL COLD ENFLEURAGE WITH FAT

This project is closest to the traditional cold enfleurage method pioneered in seventeeth-century France. It can be done in one of two ways. The first option is most like the traditional French method. The second option of using a large container, such as catering steam trays, is a recent innovation that allows easier extraction of either very large, very small, or very fragile flowers.

The project is executed in four stages. First, you'll extract the scent from the flowers into the pomade (for solid perfumes, balms, or body butters, you can stop here and use the fresh pomade immediately). To further process the enfleurage into a liquid form, you then wash the pomade with alcohol, agitating it to separate the scent from the fat by either hand or mechanical means. Next, the alcohol is purified by freezing and filtering it. The final part of the process is optional, to refine the product by extracting the absolute oil from the alcohol.

STAGE ONE: EXTRACTING THE SCENT FROM THE FLOWERS

Depending on the size of the flowers that you're working with, you can use one of two methods to perform the extraction. If the flowers are small to medium, choose the traditional cold process method. If the flowers are either large or, conversely, extremely tiny, see the note on the next page for the large-volume cold process method. This method most closely approximates the traditional French enfleurage process.

MATERIALS AND EQUIPMENT

Fat, such as deodorized coconut shortening, non-hydrogenated vegetable shortening, or shea butter

Tray or plate

Flexible or offset spatula

Knife or other scoring tool

Botanical material

Tweezers (optional)

Toothpick

Labels and recordkeeping tools

Storage jar

PROCESS

1. Spread the fat onto the tray or plate to a depth of ½ inch (1.3 cm) using a flexible spatula or an offset or angled spatula.
   OR
   Gently warm the fat to make it pourable, then pour the melted fat onto the tray or plate to a depth of ½ inch (1.3 cm).
2. If your fat is too soft at room temperature, add a small amount of beeswax now (see "Adding Beeswax to Fat" on page 70). You may want to chill the fat in the refrigerator to accelerate the solidification. Be careful if your fridge has any strong food odors because the fat will readily pick up that scent.
3. Provide more surface area for the scent molecules to adhere by scoring the solidified fat in a crisscross pattern using a knife or the edge of a spatula. Make the scores about 2 inches (5 cm) apart, to a depth of ¼ inch (6 mm).
4. Lay the prepared flowers on the fat, gently pressing them to the surface just enough to make good contact with, but not into, the fat. Optional: Use an offset spatula to spread fat onto the inside of the lid to optimize scent capture. See photo on page 69.
5. Cover the enfleurage so that foreign matter can't get into it, but not so that it's airtight; you don't want to invite mold. Place the enfleurage in a cool, dry place, away from heat or sun. If the room temperature is too warm, consider refrigerating the enfleurage.
6. Check periodically to see whether the flowers are overly wilted, no longer give off any scent, or begin to give off a less pleasant scent. Remove them when this occurs. You may need tweezers to remove pieces of the flower or pollen that remain stuck to the fat. You must do this to avoid any rotting flower bits, which will create mold on the pomade and ruin the scent.

(continued)

STAGE ONE: EXTRACTING THE SCENT FROM THE FLOWERS (CONT.)

7. Replace the flowers for as many recharges as you feel are necessary for the fat to obtain the scent strength you desire. To test the scent, use a toothpick inserted into the fat to pull a small sample. Caution: To avoid contamination, never touch the fat with your bare hands. Each time you recharge the corps, make a record of it in your notes. Be sure to include the plant names (both common and botanical), the type and amount of fat (leaf lard, vegetable shortening, and such), and the date.
8. When the fat is saturated with scent, scrape it with a spatula (this is now your pomade!) from the tray or plate and/or lid, if you coated the inside of the lid, and place it in a jar. Pack the pomade into the jar, pressing down to remove as many air pockets as you can.
9. If you're making solid perfumes, balms, or body butters, you don't need to further process the pomade; you can use it immediately (though check page 87 for tips on safely prepping it for these perfumed products). Seal the jar tightly, and label it with the plant names (common and botanical), the fat used, the number of charges, and the date. Refrigerate the pomade (preferred), or store it in a cool, dark place. See "Storing Your Enfleurage Pomades and Extraits" on page 71 for more details.
10. If you'd like to further process the pomade to extract the concentrated scent molecules for liquid perfumes, continue on to Stage Two on the next page.

NOTE: If your flowers are too large, follow these modifications for a large-container enfleurage project. Stainless steel steamer pans, like those used for catering, are my preferred containers for this process, though you can also use large glass jars with tight-fitting lids. First, place the fat into the melting pot and gently warm it until it liquefies. Remember to add beeswax if you're doing this in a warm climate or during hot weather. Pour the fat into the large enfleurage container and, if using jars, gently rotate the jar to coat the inside with a layer of the fat. Let it sit until the remaining fat that settles to the bottom of the container cools and hardens. If you choose, you can cover the inside of the catering pan lid using an offset spatula to spread some of the fat onto the lid to a depth of ¼ to ½ inch (6 to 13 mm). Then simply follow the rest of the steps.

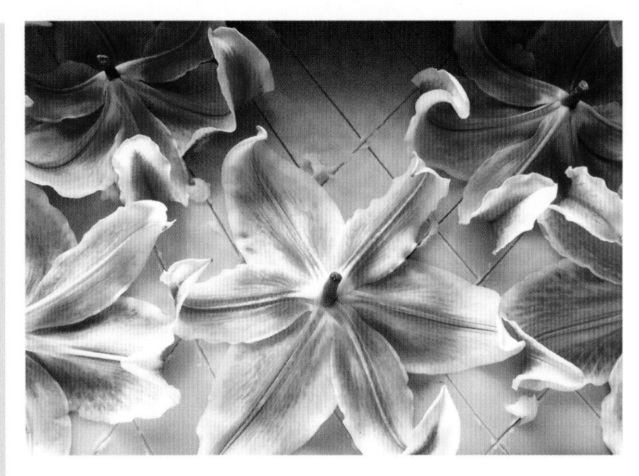

Shown here are large stargazer lilies on scored pomade.

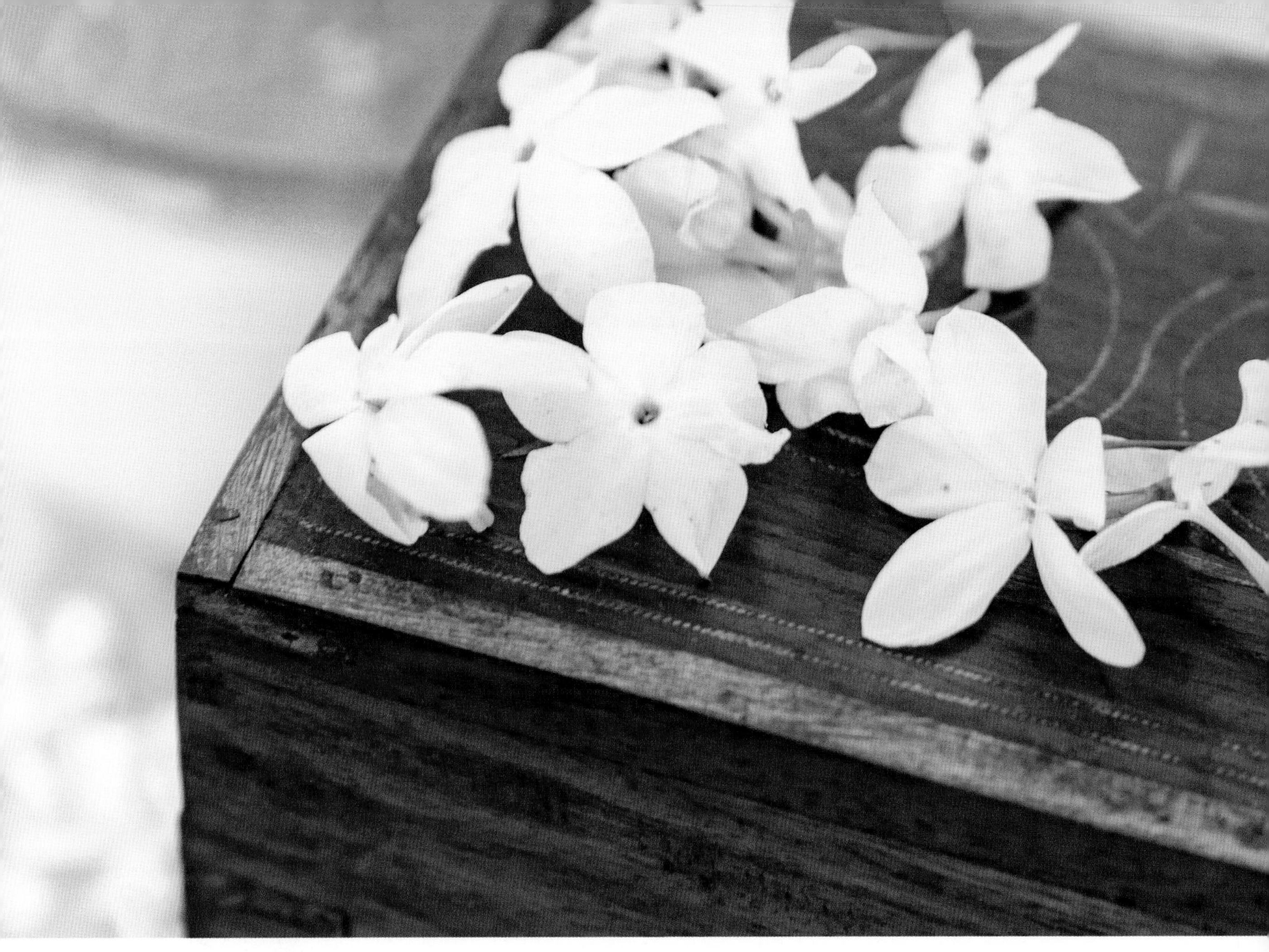

French jasmine (Jasminum grandiflorum) *flowers are rare and produce one of the best fragrances. They are also wonderfully easy to grow.*

STAGE TWO: WASHING THE POMADE

To extract the scent molecules from the pomade for use in perfumes, it's necessary to wash the pomade with alcohol, either mechanically or by hand. This releases the scent molecules from the fat into the alcohol. Both the pomade and the extrait can be reprocessed, as follows. After the first washing, the pomade can be rewashed up to two more times, using fresh alcohol for each wash. The first washing results in the strongest extrait, so you could choose to stop the extraction process here. Additionally, you can choose to strengthen the extrait with recharges of more pomade. Each wash is typically for 5 to 10 days. Following these washes, the pomade still retains some scent, so it can be used in soaps and other cosmetics, such as creams and lotions. It is not necessary to measure the alcohol and pomade precisely, but traditionally, the washes are done using an equal weight or volume of pomade and alcohol.

MANUAL COLD WASHING METHOD

The manual method of washing pomade in a jar is the least time-consuming, but it's also the least efficient method for extracting the scent molecules into the alcohol. However, it's an easy way to get experience with the process, and you may wish to experiment to observe the results. Note that the washing jar's capacity must be at least twice the volume of the pomade that you're washing. So, if you're going to wash 16 ounces (473 ml) of pomade, you'll need a quart (945-ml) jar to accommodate the matching amount of alcohol.

MATERIALS AND EQUIPMENT

Scented pomade

Spatula or spoon

Airtight, sanitized jars for processing and/or storing the pomade

Chopstick

190-proof alcohol

Labels and record-keeping tools

Glass or stainless steel funnel

Filter papers

PROCESS

1. From the original pomade container, using a spatula or spoon to scoop the pomade, fill the processing jar about halfway. Do not pack it tightly because air spaces are required for this process.
2. Break the pomade into small pieces. If you need to, use an implement such as a chopstick or spoon to do this (but not your fingers).
3. Add a volume of alcohol equal to the volume of the pomade, and immediately screw the jar lid on tightly. Label the jar with the name of the pomade, type and strength of alcohol used, the number of pomade charges, and the date.
4. Shake the jar vigorously every hour, if possible. The alcohol will begin to break up the pieces of pomade. The goal is to make the pomade and alcohol into a slurry.
5. Continue shaking the jar as often as possible, for at least 5—and up to 10—days. Your nose will tell you that you've pulled all the scent you can get from the fat when the scent no longer grows stronger.
6. Pour the alcohol and pomade slurry through a funnel lined with filter paper and press with a spoon to force the alcohol through. You can gently squeeze the filter after to remove more alcohol. Save the leftover pomade in a jar for other uses.
7. If you wish to make recharges of the alcohol by adding new pomade, repeat steps 1 through 5 until the strength of the scent is satisfactory to you, or until you have no more pomade to wash. Keep a record of the number of washes or recharges you do.
8. To process the scented alcohol further and produce a more clarified and concentrated product (recommended), continue on to Stage Three on page 83.
9. Alternatively, you can use this scented alcohol as is if you'd like. Make sure to label the jar with the pomade name, fat used, number of pomade charges, type and strength of alcohol used, number of washing charges, and the date. Refrigerate the extrait (preferred), or store it in a cool, dark place. See "Storing Your Enfleurage Pomades and Extraits" on page 71 for more plant- and solvent-specific storage details. Reserve the used pomade for other purposes if you'd like (see page 87 to safely prepare it for your perfumed products).

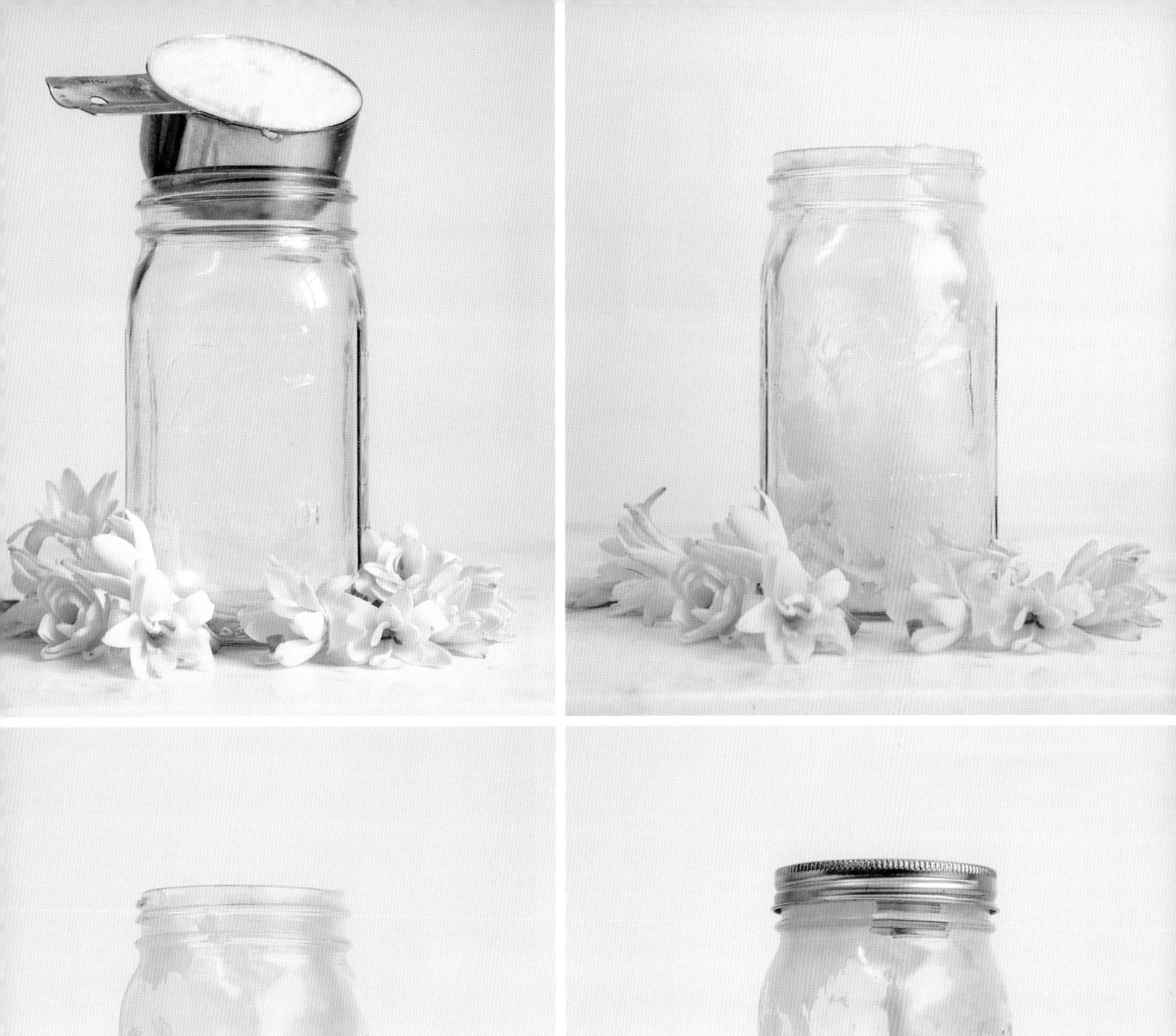
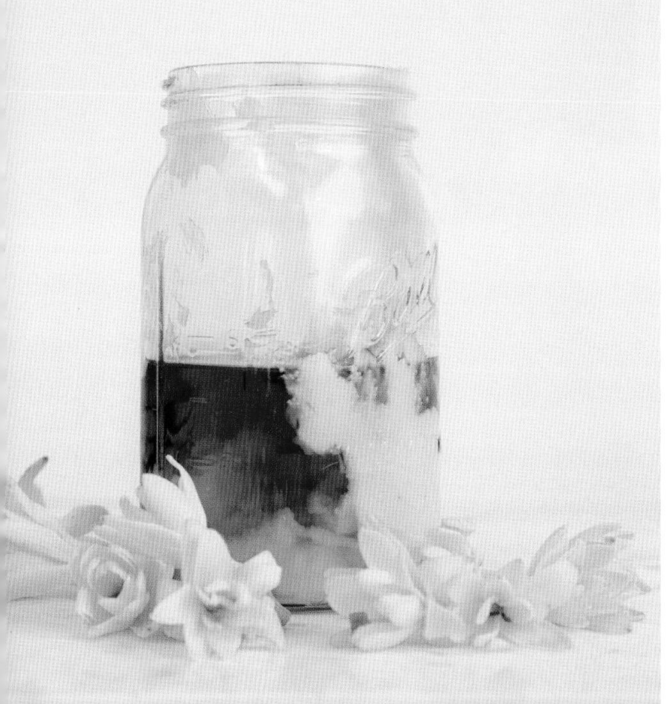
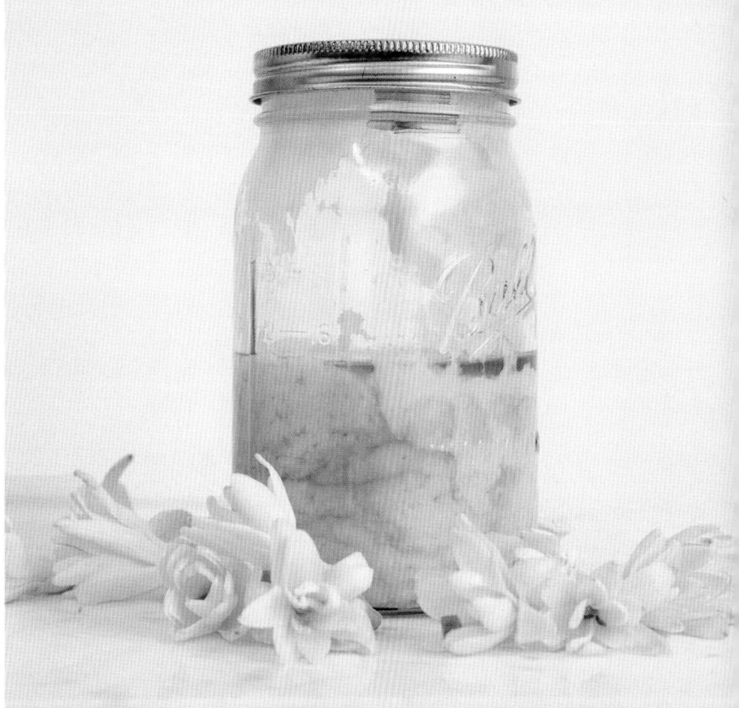

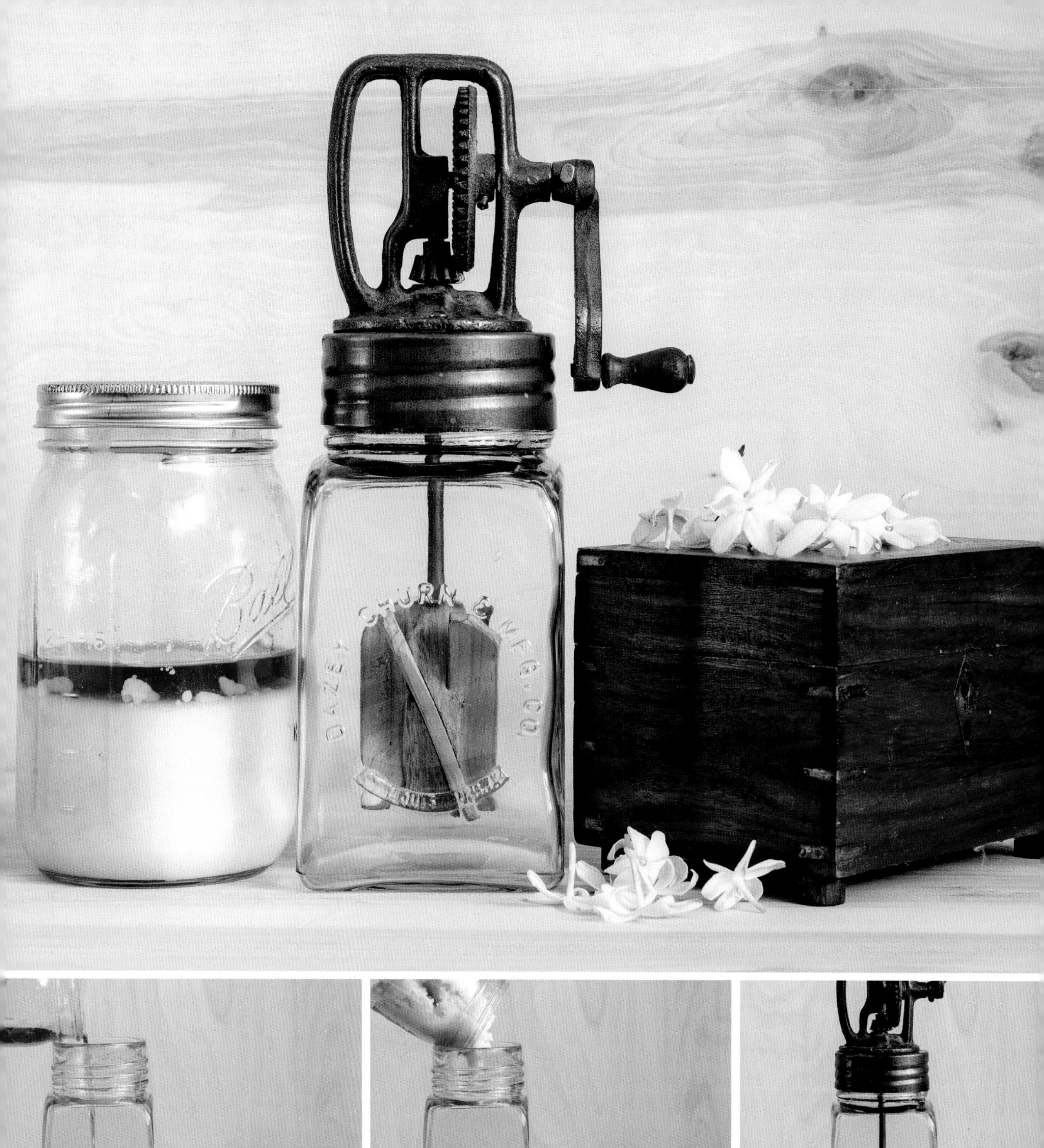
Ball
DAZEY CHURN & MFG. CO.

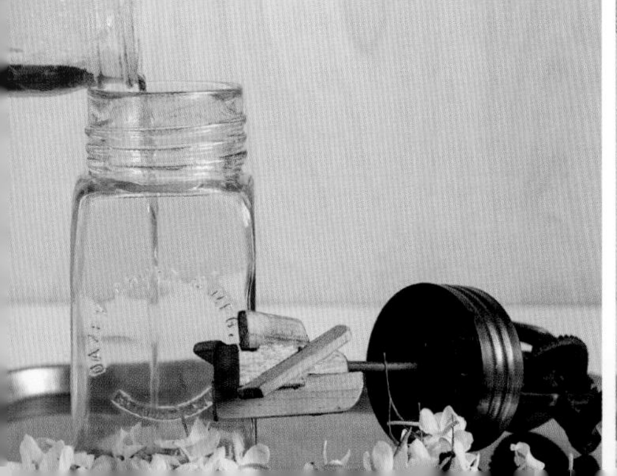

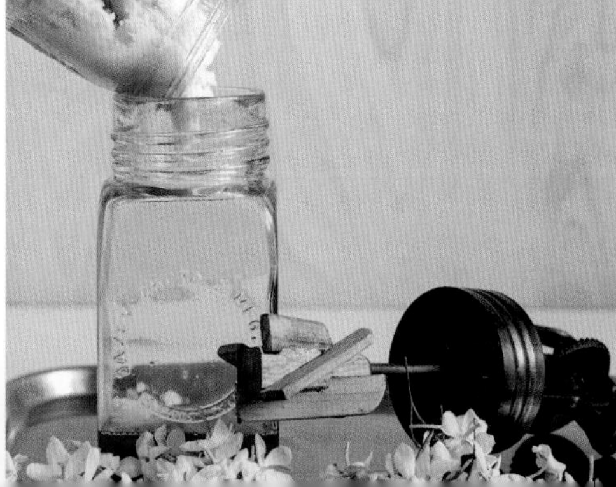

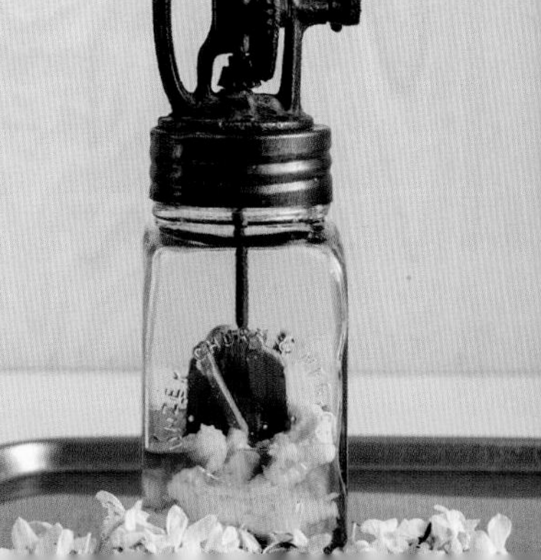

MECHANICAL COLD WASHING METHOD

Traditionally, pomades were washed by a mechanical process that vigorously stirred the fat for days in a machine called a *batteuse*, an enclosed container with a motor-driven central rod with extending arms to stir the pomade and alcohol combination. The agitation separated the oil from the fat, transferring it to the alcohol. My updated method calls for improvising a batteuse by using several objects to wash the pomade. I encourage you to try this as well. You may discover something effective, low-cost, and easy for you to manage. A simple kitchen stand mixer works very well for an improvised, modern batteuse, so I've written the instructions for a stand mixer. The original batteuses were lined with tin and had wooden paddles. I have a small, hand-cranked glass butter churn with wooden paddles that I use while I'm outside relaxing in the garden or sitting watching TV. It's a bit meditative, if noisy. Electric butter churns are available, and you might consider one if you plan to process a lot of pomade.

MATERIALS AND EQUIPMENT

Stand mixer or butter churn (optional)

Scented pomade

190-proof alcohol

Measuring cups of varying sizes (optional)

Labels and record-keeping tools

Spoon or flexible spatula

Glass or stainless steel funnel

Filter papers

Airtight jars for processing and/or storing the pomade

PROCESS

1. If you're using a stand mixer, position the beaters so that you can mark where they would penetrate the lid once they're attached to the mixer. (See the discussion about non-planetary kitchen stand mixers on page 69.) Cut two small slits in the plastic lid where the beaters will go.
2. Insert the beaters in the slits, and tape the slits shut to minimize evaporation.
3. Using the measuring cup, measure and place equal amounts of the pomade and alcohol in the bowl, lower the beaters and lid, and snap the lid on securely. Start the motor on a slow speed.
4. Run the motor on a slow speed for at least one day, or longer, if you prefer.
5. Check your mixer and the pomade and alcohol blend in the bowl periodically to be certain that it's making a slurry. If necessary, use a spoon or spatula to scrape pomade from the side of the bowl. Since we're in uncharted, experimental territory of a modern-day batteuse here, let your instincts be your guide. Also, be conscious of the mixer because some motors can only run for a certain amount of time before they need to cool down.
6. Pour the alcohol/pomade slurry through a funnel lined with filter papers into a sanitized jar and screw the lid on immediately. This step may take some time; you can press the slurry with a spoon to speed the alcohol extraction.

(continued)

MECHANICAL COLD WASHING METHOD (CONT.)

7. Your nose will tell you when you've pulled all the scent you can get from the fat because you will no longer find the scent growing stronger each time you smell it.
8. If you wish to recharge the alcohol by adding new pomade, repeat steps 3 through 7 until the strength of the scent is satisfactory to you, or until you have no more pomade to wash. Keep a record of the number of charges or washes you do.
9. Pour the alcohol into a sanitized jar, and immediately place the lid on tightly. Label the jar with all pertinent information, including the plant names (common and botanical), type and strength of alcohol, the number of corps charges, and the bottling date.
10. To process the scented alcohol further and produce a more clarified and concentrated product (recommended), continue on to Stage Three on page 83.
11. Alternatively, you can use this scented alcohol as is if you'd like. Make sure to label the jar and either refrigerate the extrait (preferred) or store it in a cool, dark place. See "Storing Your Enfleurage Pomades and Extraits" on page 71 for more plant- and solvent-specific storage details. Reserve the used pomade for other purposes if you'd like (see page 87 to safely prepare it for your perfumed products).

HOT WASHING METHOD

This method of extraction is particularly effective when the pomade contains beeswax. Heating the pomade and alcohol helps to break the bond between the scent molecules and the wax. The scent bonds with the alcohol, and as the solution cools, the fat precipitates out, leaving behind the scented alcohol.

Before you begin this process, you need to do some planning. First, decide how much extrait you want to make. It's easiest to do this in a "round number" amount, such as 100 milliliters. Then determine how much pomade you have, and how many washings you will do. For example, if you have four times the volume of pomade to volume of extrait you wish to make, you'll make four washes, using one-quarter of the pomade for each washing.

MATERIALS AND EQUIPMENT

190-proof alcohol

500-ml or larger beaker (as determined by amount you are processing) or non-reactive pot

Pomade

Canning jar with disk lid (don't use ring to tighten lid during processing)

Heat source (electric cup warmer, hot plate, or electric stove top)

Thermometer

Stainless steel or glass funnel

Filter papers

Labels and record-keeping tools

PROCESS

1. Measure the alcohol into the beaker.
2. Add the pomade to the alcohol in the beaker.
3. Pour the mixture into the canning jar.
4. Place the jar on your chosen heat source. You can use an electric cup warmer for up to 8 ounces (236 ml) of pomade, or a hot plate for larger amounts of pomade, up to 64 ounces (2 L).
5. Heat the alcohol and pomade to 86 to 104°F (30 to 40°C). This is the safest heat range to dissolve the fat (and any wax needed if you live in a warm climate) and to allow the scent molecules to move into solution with the alcohol. If the mixture rises above this temperature, it increases the likelihood of the alcohol igniting, and causes evaporation diffusing into the air and wasting some of the precious scent you worked hard to extract.

CAUTION: If you're using a canning jar for this process, do not use the ring to tighten the lid during the processing; otherwise, you risk explosion from a buildup of pressure and the alcohol.

6. Use a thermometer to monitor the temperature closely until the fat is dissolved, as well as any wax. Once everything is melted together, allow the mixture to completely cool.

(continued)

HOT WASHING METHOD (CONT.)

7. Put the vessel, with the cover or lid still in place, into a freezer. Cool the contents to 32°F (0°C) or lower, and maintain that temperature for at least 12 hours. The fat (and any wax) will sink to the bottom.
8. Use a stainless steel or glass funnel with three coffee filters to carefully decant the alcohol from the top of the jar into a clean storage jar. Press the fat with a spoon to release more extrait, then gather the filters at the top and gently squeeze to release more extrait. Save the pomade for other uses. Filter the fat (and any wax) from the bottom of the first jar, adding the recovered alcohol to the jar containing the decanted extrait. Immediately place the lid on tightly.
9. To process the scented alcohol further and produce a more clarified and concentrated product (recommended), continue onto Stage Three on page 83.
10. Alternatively, you can use this scented alcohol as is if you'd like. Make sure to label the jar with the pomade name, fat used, number of pomade charges, type and strength of alcohol used, number of washing charges, and the date. Refrigerate the extrait (preferred), or store it in a cool, dark place. See "Storing Your Enfleurage Pomades and Extraits" on page 71 for more plant- and solvent-specific storage details. Reserve the used pomade for other purposes if you'd like (see page 87 to safely prepare it for your perfumed products).

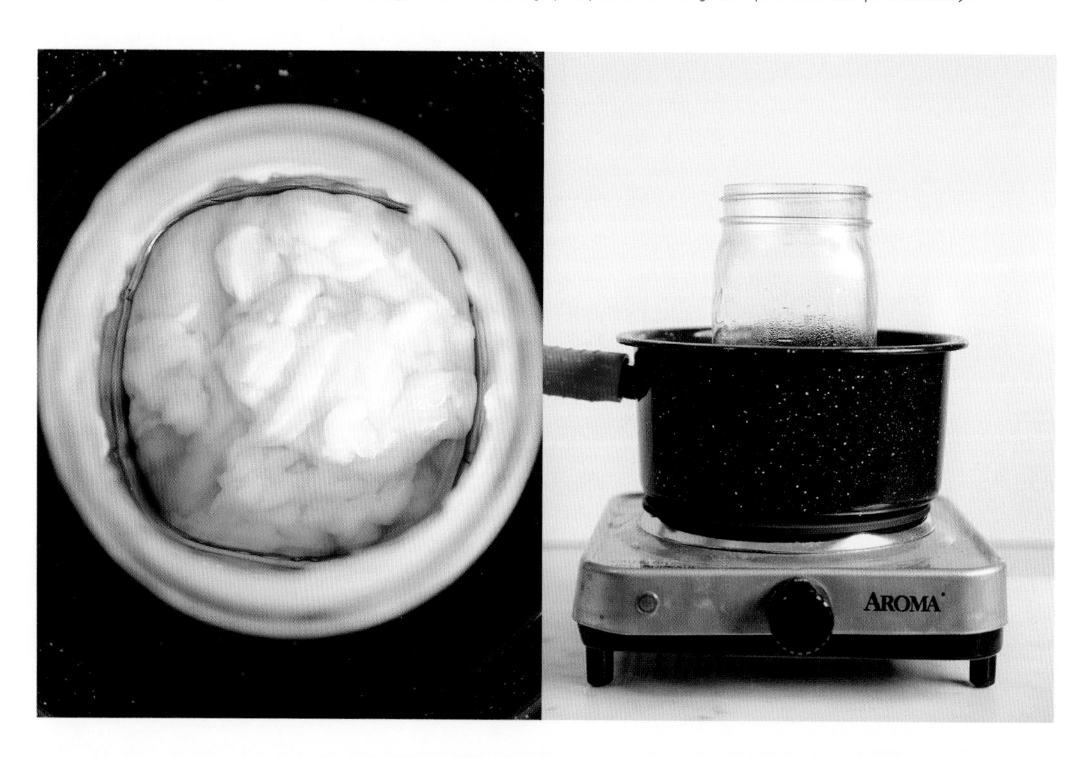

STAGE THREE: CLARIFYING THE EXTRAIT

After washing the pomade, you can process the extrait to separate the scented alcohol from any residual fat by freezing and filtering it. I highly recommend doing this simple step, as it will give you an exceptionally clear and high-quality product.

MATERIALS AND EQUIPMENT

Alcohol extrait and pomade

Stainless steel mesh strainer or glass or stainless steel funnel

Jar with a tight-fitting lid

3 coffee filter papers

190-proof alcohol

Stainless steel spoon

Labels and record-keeping tools

PROCESS

1. Place the jar containing the washed alcohol extrait in the freezer for at least 24 hours. If you followed the Hot Washing Method on page 81, you are now freezing the alcohol for a second time. This step allows any heavier dissolved fat molecules that may be suspended in the alcohol to fall to the bottom of the liquid. It may be about 50/50 liquid to pomade.
2. Place the strainer or funnel over a jar that you will use to store the extrait.
3. Pre-wet the filter papers with 190-proof alcohol and place them into the strainer or funnel.
4. Carefully decant the clear alcohol portion of the extrait into the filter, leaving any settled fat at the bottom of the original jar.
5. Then, carefully pour the semi-liquid pomade into the filter, and press down with a stainless steel spoon to help release more extrait. After releasing as much extrait as you can with the spoon, gather up the top filter paper into a pouch, pinching the top shut, and gently squeeze out as much extrait as possible. You should have a firm piece of pomade left after this. Put it in a jar, cover the jar and save it for another perfume project, like a solid perfume.
6. Screw the lid of the jar of clarified extrait on tightly and label it, using all of the information from Stage Two: the pomade name, fat used, number of pomade charges, type and strength of alcohol used, number of washing charges, and the date.

(continued)

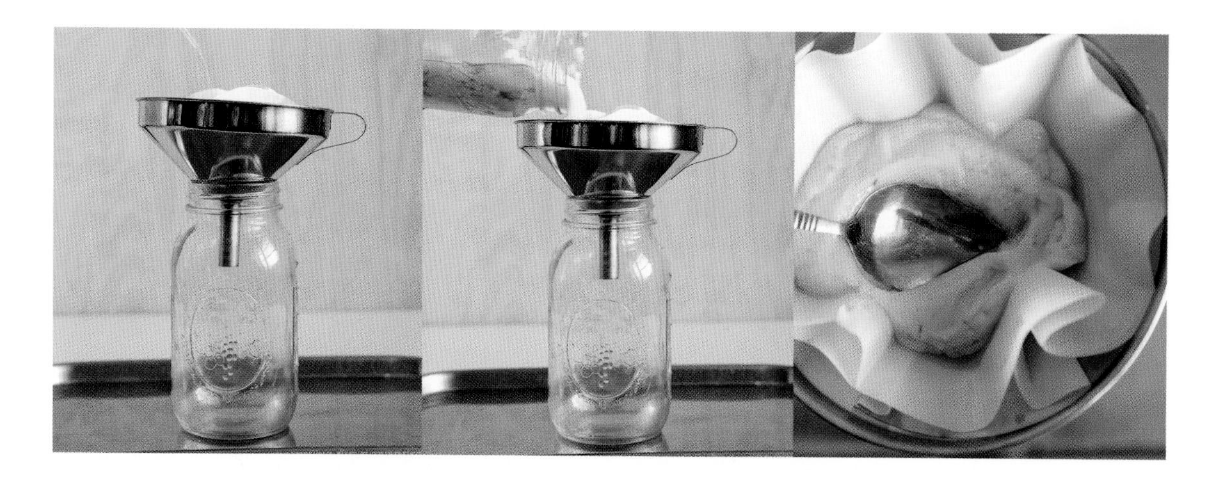

STAGE THREE: CLARIFYING THE EXTRAIT (CONT.)

7. Store in a cool, dark, dry place, or refrigerate it, for future use. See "Storing Your Enfleurage Pomades and Extraits" on page 71 for more plant- and solvent-specific storage details.

8. Congratulations! You are now the proud creator of an ancient form of perfume ingredient that was regarded with the highest esteem throughout history by the most accomplished perfume makers. This clarified alcohol extrait can now be used to make perfume in several different ways. You can use it at full strength in a perfume formula, or you can choose to use it as part of the total alcohol in a formula. You can also use it in diluted, smaller quantities to give what is called a "sheer" note to the perfume—a lightly scented addition. And finally, you can use it as a component, such as a top, middle, or base note—either as a stand-alone note or in a blended accord of scents that make up the top, middle, or base of a perfume. (These components are described in Chapter 5.)

9. However, if you choose, you can process the extrait further by extracting the scented absolute oil from it. The absolute oil remains clear, even when the temperature is cold, and provides a rich, strong scent to your perfume. Continue on to the final step, Stage Four, on the next page.

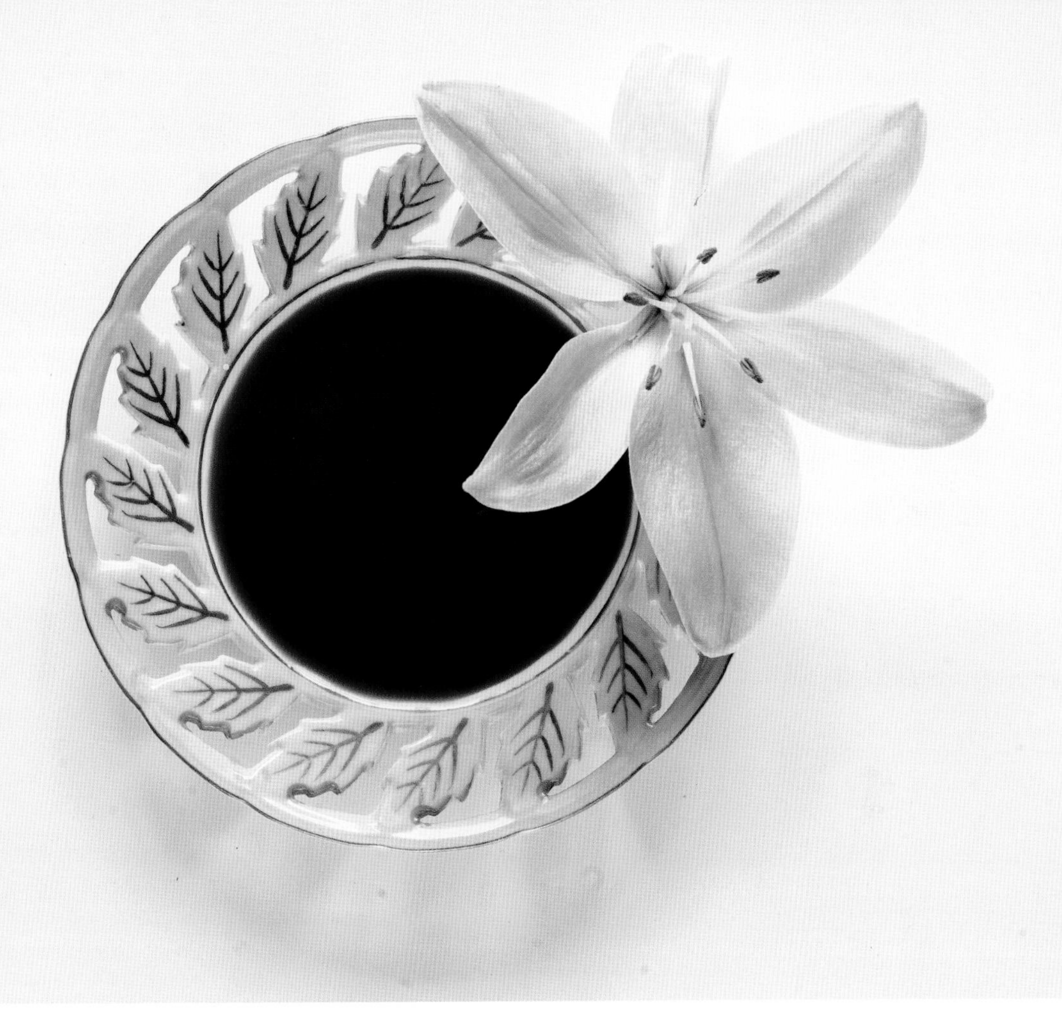

When you are using the low-tech method to evaporate the alcohol from the extrait, you'll find some variations in color and also the nature of the absolute left behind. Sometimes it will be light, sometimes dark and opaque, depending upon your original extrait.

STAGE FOUR: EXTRACTING THE ABSOLUTE OIL

If you choose to refine your extrait further to produce an absolute oil, you can use either the low-tech evaporation method or the high-tech method of vacuum distillation, and you will be rewarded with a rare and beautiful oil. With either process, the absolute oil that you obtain is more concentrated, so you will lose quite a bit of volume. Besides the experimental thrill, an advantage of making the absolute oil is that it works well in both oil- and alcohol-based perfumes.

LOW-TECH ABSOLUTE OIL EXTRACTION

Technically in traditional French perfumery, only vacuum distillation yields absolute oil. We home perfumers can approximate this using a low-tech evaporation method. I've used this method for years to evaporate the alcohol from enfleurage extrait, yielding a product very similar to an absolute oil. The evaporation process is done outdoors to prevent a buildup of alcohol vapors, which can be flammable. Experiment first, using only a small amount of extrait, so that you don't lose all of your extrait if there is an accident, or you make a mistake while you're learning how to do this. (See page 85 for a photo showing this method.)

MATERIALS AND EQUIPMENT

Clarified, scented alcohol extrait

Nonreactive deep plate, or shallow jar

Cheesecloth, muslin, or other breathable cloth

Spatula or small stainless steel spoon

Vial or small jar

Labels and record-keeping tools

PROCESS

NOTE: Because of the nature of this process, you will likely lose some of the top notes during evaporation. These are the most volatile—the first fleeting notes that you smell. It's best to perform the extraction on a dry day with low humidity because you can lose more of the top notes in high humidity.

1. Pour the extrait into your chosen evaporation receptacle.
2. Suspend or drape the cloth cover over the container in such a way that it doesn't fall into the extrait.

TIP: If you decide to use a shallow jar for evaporation, it's a good idea to use a Mason-type canning jar with a ring lid, which you can screw over the cloth cover to hold it in place and keep small bugs out. If the container is larger, secure the cloth with a rubber band, or tuck the cloth underneath.

3. Place the container in an outdoor place, protected from rain. Make sure it's away from any open flame or a spot where it might be knocked over.
4. Check the extrait the following day to see whether it's ready. It should be reduced in volume and look thick and syrupy. When the alcohol evaporates, it leaves very little absolute oil, but it's highly concentrated.
5. After the alcohol evaporates from the extrait, use a spatula or spoon to scrape the absolute oil from the evaporation vessel and put it into a vial or small jar with a tight-fitting cap or lid.
6. Label the bottle with the plant names (common and botanical), fat used, number of flower charges, number of pomade washes, and the final bottling date. Store in a cool, dark place. See "Storing Your Enfleurage Pomades and Extraits" on page 71 for more plant- and solvent-specific storage details.

HIGH-TECH ABSOLUTE OIL EXTRACTION—VACUUM DISTILLATION

Vacuum distillation is one way to extract the absolute oil from the scented alcohol after its separation from the pomade fat or enfleurage oil (see "Vacuum Distillation" on page 53). The alcohol is distilled with low heat and low pressure, using an additional piece of equipment called a vacuum column. If you have a distillation unit with a vacuum column, you can use it to distill the alcohol, leaving behind the absolute oil. Not all distillation units accept the addition of a vacuum column, so check with the manufacturer if this is something you wish to pursue.

When you evaporate the alcohol using this process, the absolute oil that it yields is of the highest quality of any extraction that you will make in this book. The absolute oil is extremely concentrated and highly desirable for use in fine perfumery. It can be used as an absolute when you blend your fragrances, or added directly to oil, body butters, and other fragrant products.

Note: Always remember that alcohol vapors are flammable. Take appropriate precautions if you choose to further process your extrait using this method, which involves heat.

PREPARING PROCESSED POMADE FOR PRODUCTS

After pomade is washed, it still retains scent. Because of this, you can use it in solid perfumes, body butters, soaps, and some hair preparations. Before using the pomade for these purposes, one final process removes any residual alcohol from it. Note that in soap making, residual alcohol in pomade could cause the soap to "trace," or thicken, more quickly, or even to seize, so be especially vigilant when you use it for this.

MATERIALS AND EQUIPMENT

Pomade

Stainless steel tray or nonreactive plate or dish

Spoon or spatula

Clean towel or paper

Labels and record-keeping tools

Sterilized container

PROCESS

1. After filtering, scrape the pomade from the filters using a spoon or spatula. Spread the used pomade in a thin layer on a nonreactive surface, such as a stainless steel tray.
2. Cover the tray with a clean towel or paper to keep dust and insects away from the pomade.
3. Set the tray in a cool, dry place and allow the small amount of remaining alcohol to evaporate. It may take a few hours. You may stir it occasionally to expose more surface area to evaporation.
4. Store the finished pomade in a properly labeled container in a cool, dark, dry place.

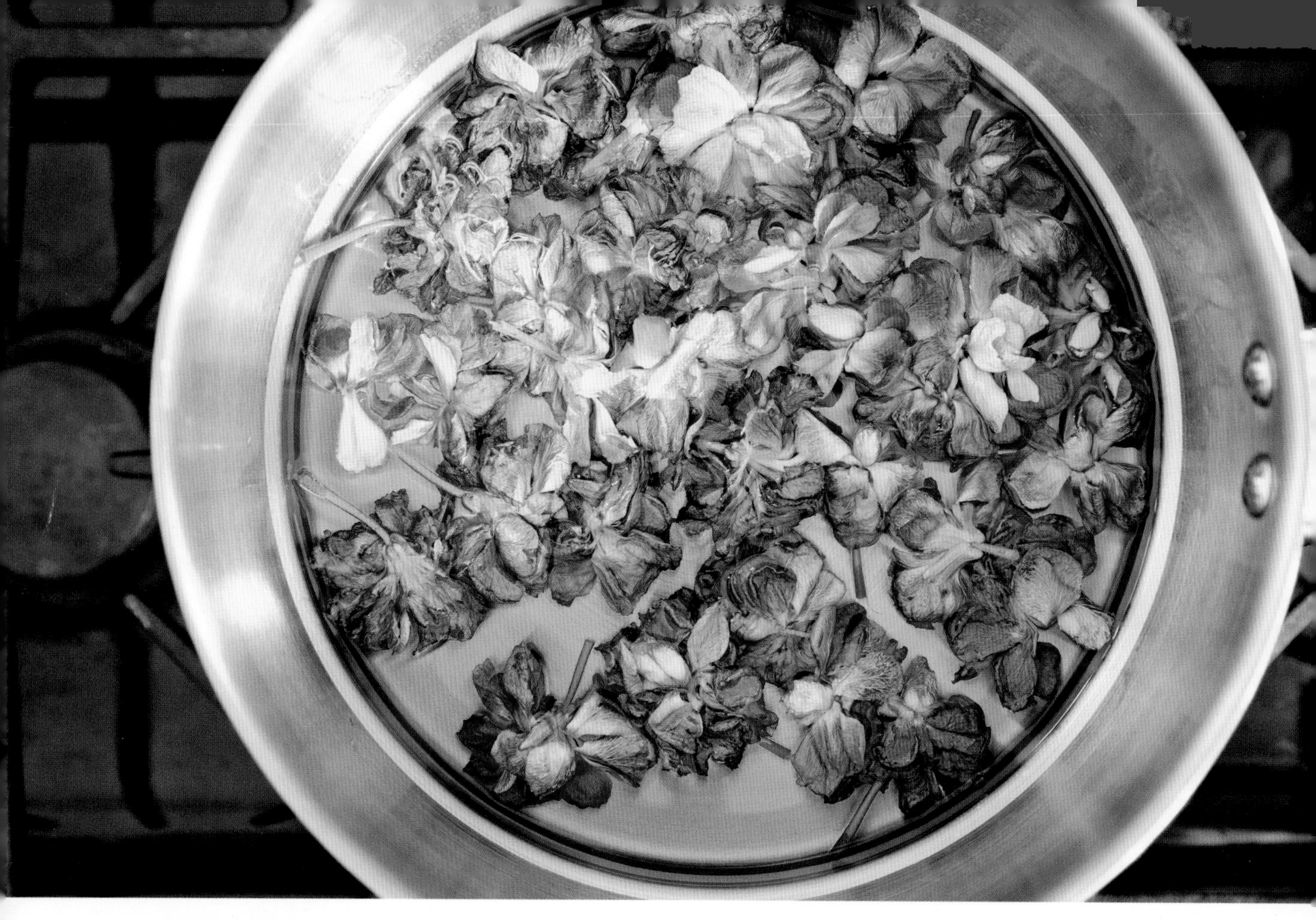

Delicate flowers are easy to process for scent extraction using the French method of hot maceration. Shown here are night-scented stocks. Recharge as necessary to obtain the desired scent strength. The scented oil can be used as is, or further processed to obtain an extrait or absolute.

HOT ENFLEURAGE: MACERATION

Maceration is an enfleurage method in which the scent is extracted from flowers using heated fat or oil, and in perfumery, this is the traditional French process of enfleurage in hot oil, not to be confused with hot infusion. Some flowers aren't suitable for distillation or cold enfleurage, and others flowers are too fragile for pomade enfleurage because they will fall apart, as orange blossoms tend to do, or get stuck in the fat. Maceration is only used for delicate flowers, such as roses, violets, cassie (mimosa), orange flowers, lily of the valley, and similar delicate flowers you may have. This method is quick and gives lovely results. A tiny bit of the top notes is lost because of the heat, but if you have a lot of flowers and want to process them quickly, maceration wins over traditional cold enfleurage in pomade. The most commonly used oils are moringa oil (historically called ben oil) and light olive oil because they don't spoil as quickly as most other oils.

You will go through several steps to process the flowers, much as you do for cold process enfleurage: first extracting the scent from the flowers in heated oil, recharging as many times as needed, and then either using the oil as is or further processing it to create an alcohol extrait or, finally, an absolute oil.

STAGE ONE: EXTRACTING THE SCENT FROM THE FLOWERS

Historically, with the French hot enfleurage method, flowers are combined with fat, heated, and stirred for several hours before the flowers are removed and replaced with fresh ones, and that's what we'll be doing here. This process is repeated several times until the fat is sufficiently scented.

MATERIALS AND EQUIPMENT

Oil or fat, such as moringa or light olive, enough to cover the flowers

Nonreactive pan (glass, stainless steel) of sufficient size to hold the solvent and flowers

Heating unit of your choice: slow cooker or stove top/hot plate (for use with double boiler)

Flowers

Spoon

Thermometer

Nonreactive strainer

Clean bowl or jar

Toothpick or scent strip

Sanitized jar

Labels and record-keeping tools

PROCESS

1. Place the oil or fat into the nonreactive pan.
2. Place the pan onto the heating surface and add the flowers to it, making sure there is enough solvent to cover the flowers.
3. Slowly warm the oil or fat to within the temperature range of 140 to 158°F (60 to 70°C).
4. Gently stir the solvent and flowers frequently, monitoring the temperature with a thermometer if needed.
5. After a few hours, or as soon as they become translucent or limp, no longer give off any scent, or begin to give off a less pleasant scent, strain the spent flowers through a nonreactive strainer into a clean bowl or jar.
6. Recharge the solvent with fresh flowers, repeating as many times as you feel are necessary for the fat to obtain the scent strength you desire. To test the scent, use a toothpick or scent strip inserted into the oil or fat to pull a small sample. Caution: To avoid contamination, never touch the fat with your bare hands. Each time you recharge the solvent, make a record of it in your notes. Be sure to include the plant names (both common and botanical), the type and amount of fat, and the date.
7. When the oil is saturated with scent, strain it into a sanitized jar and allow it to cool. Label the jar with the name, oil or fat used, number of charges, and the date. This scented oil or fat can now be used in oil perfumes, massage oils, soaps and body butters! If you're not using it right away, tightly put the lid on and store in a cool, dark place. See "Storing Your Enfleurage Pomades and Extraits" on page 71 for more details.
8. If you'd like to further process the scented pomade oil to extract the concentrated scent molecules for alcohol perfumes, continue on to Stage Two on page 91.

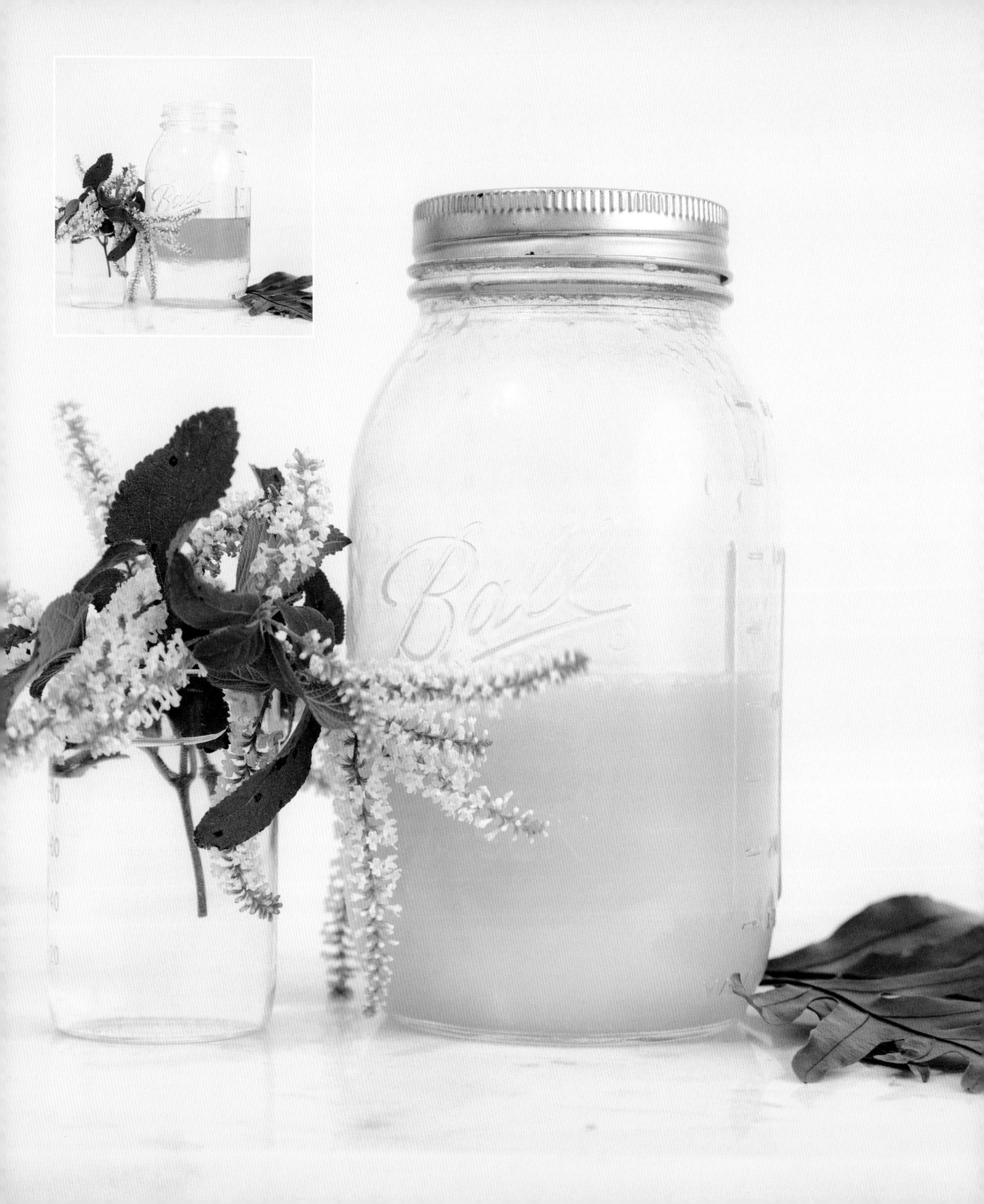
Ball

STAGE TWO: WASHING THE ENFLEURAGE OIL

After extraction, as in the cold process method, the oil is washed with alcohol to transfer the oil's scent to the alcohol, creating a more concentrated and versatile extrait.

MATERIALS AND EQUIPMENT

Scented pomade oil

Butter churn or stand mixer (optional)

190-proof alcohol

Airtight, sanitized jars

Pipette (optional)

Labels and record-keeping tools

PROCESS

1. Wash the oil with your preferred method. See page 76 for instructions and photos for manual cold washing—the fastest and easiest, but least effective. See page 79 for instructions and photos for mechanical washing—slower and requiring a stand mixer or butter churn, but the most effective. Wash the oil with alcohol at a ratio of 1:1.
2. After washing, allow the oil and alcohol to sit undisturbed until there are two separate and distinct layers. Decant the alcohol into a sanitized jar. If you choose, use a pipette to draw the oil from the alcohol.
3. If needed, recharge the alcohol with fresh pomade oil until either you reach your desired scent level or you use up all of the pomade. Keep a record of the number of charges or washes you do.
4. When finished, pour the alcohol into a sanitized jar, and immediately place the lid on tight.
5. To process the scented alcohol further and produce a more clarified and concentrated product (recommended), continue onto Stage Three on page 92.
6. Alternatively, you can use this scented alcohol as is if you'd like. Label the alcohol jar with the name of the plant, plant part used, type of oil used for extraction, number of flower charges, type and strength of alcohol, and the date. Store it in a cool, dark place. See "Storing Your Enfleurage Pomades and Extraits" on page 71 for more details.
7. Reserve the used fragrant oil for use in other perfumed products. Transfer the oil to a sanitized jar, label it appropriately, and store it in a cool, dark place.

STAGE THREE: CLARIFYING THE ENFLEURAGE OIL EXTRAIT

This process separates any remaining oil (and any wax) from the alcohol extrait. This step is necessary to provide you with a clear extrait that can be used directly in perfumes, and with the oil and wax eliminated, the perfume will stay clear even when it is cold. See page 84 for photos showing an extrait being clarified.

MATERIALS AND EQUIPMENT

Alcohol extrait

Sanitized jar with a tight-fitting lid

Filter papers

Nonreactive strainer

Alcohol (190 proof recommended)

Labels and record-keeping tools

PROCESS

1. Freeze the jar of alcohol for 24 hours to let any remaining fat or wax settle to the bottom.
2. Carefully decant the alcohol into a sanitized jar, leaving the fat undisturbed at the bottom of the original jar. For a clearer extrait, place a filter paper into the strainer, pre-wet it with alcohol, and pour the alcohol extrait through the filter before decanting it into the sanitized jar.
3. Tightly screw on the lid of the jar of extrait and label it with the common and botanical names, type of fat and alcohol used, number of charges, and the date.
4. Refrigerate the alcohol extrait if you don't plan to use it right away. See "Storing Your Enfleurage Pomades and Extraits" on page 71 for more details. You can use the alcohol as is, or further process it into an absolute oil—see Stage Four on the next page.

STAGE FOUR: EXTRACTING ABSOLUTE OIL

This process evaporates the alcohol from the extrait, leaving behind the final, highest quality product—absolute oil. This absolute oil works very well in both oil-based and alcohol-based perfumes. See page 85 for a photo showing this process.

MATERIALS AND EQUIPMENT

Clarified alcohol extrait

Nonreactive deep plate, tray, or shallow vessel with a large surface area

Porous cover, such as muslin, cheesecloth, or other lightweight cloth

Spatula or other scraper

Storage bottle with a tight-fitting lid

Labels and record-keeping tools

PROCESS

1. Pour the extrait onto the plate or tray or into the shallow vessel.
2. Cover the vessel with one of the porous covers to protect it from dust, particulate matter, and bugs while the alcohol evaporates.
3. Place the container in an outdoor place, protected from rain. Make sure it's away from any open flame or a spot where it might be knocked over.
4. When the alcohol has evaporated and only the absolute oil remains, scrape it from the tray and place it into the storage bottle.
5. Label the bottle with the type of extrait, all the information from the previous stage, and the date that it was made.
6. Store the absolute oil in the refrigerator or a cool, dark place. See "Storing Your Enfleurage Pomades and Extraits" on page 71 for more details.

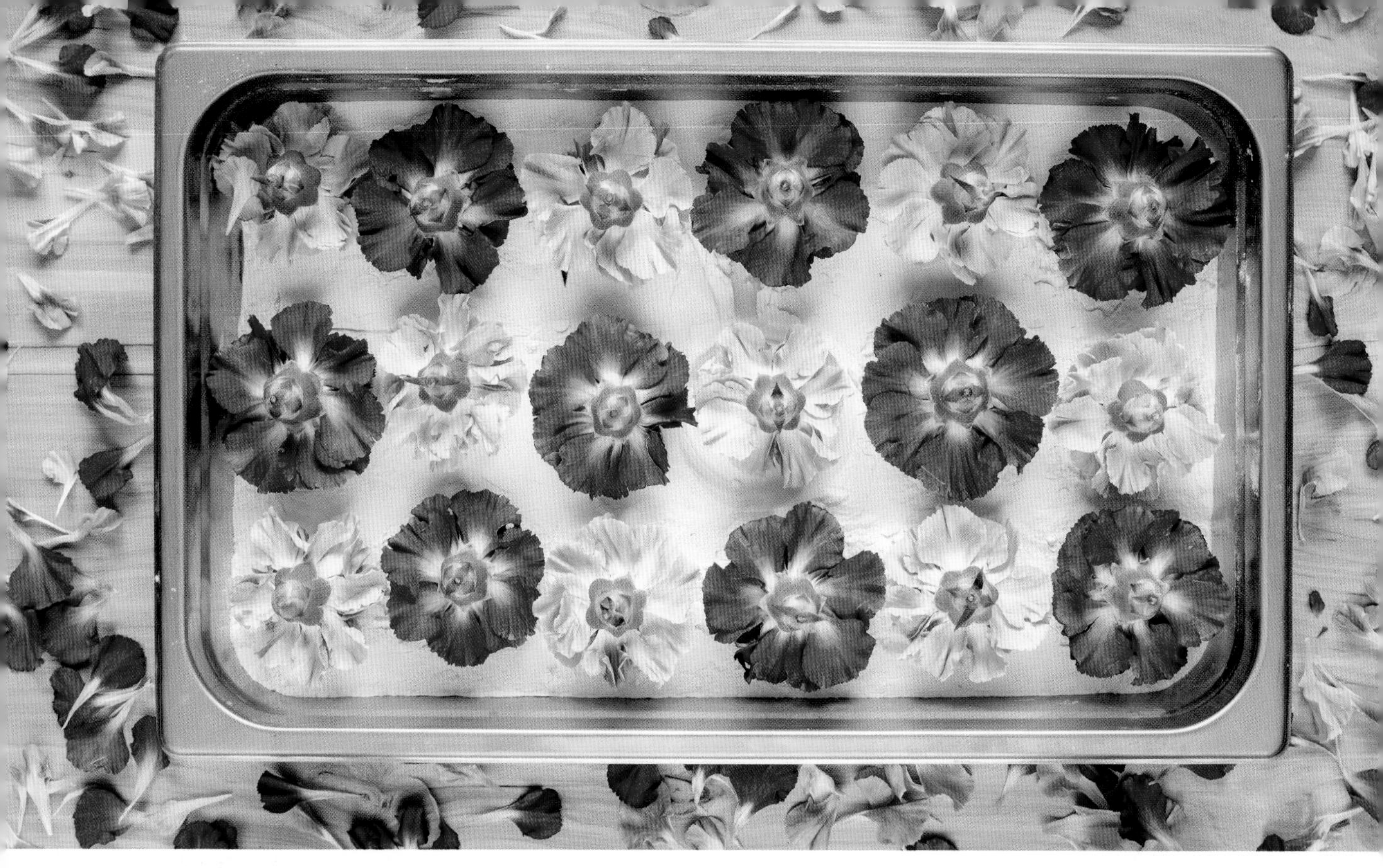

Cold powder enfleurage is so easy, and so rewarding! Some flowers that are impossible to get essential oil from—such as lilac, lily of the valley, and daphne—would yield their scents to powder, and then you can use it as body powder or deodorant powder.

ENFLEURAGE DES POUDRES: POWDER ENFLEURAGE

The process of making perfumed body powders is quite rewarding. You can make floral dusting powders that gently perfume your body, or herbal powders to use as deodorant. You can even make powders infused with exotically scented incense. Scented dusting powders (body powders) are made by exposing the powder of your choice to flowers or other scented botanical material (resins, gums, or woods), or to incense vapors. I'll give you the steps to make both cold process powders, best for flowers and leaves, and hot process powders. The hot vapor powder method is a great way to extract the scent of resins, such as frankincense and myrrh.

COLD POWDER ENFLEURAGE

This is one of the easiest projects in this book, and it enables you to make powders with flowers that don't usually release their scent well in tinctures or don't distill well, including lilac, lily of the valley, freesia, and daphne. I recommend using powders made from arrowroot, tapioca root, rice, or non-GMO cornstarch. These are the least scented and have the best "slip"—the silkiest feel. I usually use 1 pound (454 g) of flour for each enfleurage, but you can use more or less depending on how much of the botanical you have; you will be placing the botanical in a single layer, at least 2 inches (5 cm) deep, across the top of your flour in a tray.

Your scented powders will last longer if you add powdered orrisroot, or powdered ambrette seed, in small amounts to the flour because they act as fixatives. For every 14 ounces (397 g) of powder, add 2 ounces (57 g) of powdered orrisroot or ambrette seed, for a total of 16 ounces (454 g), and mix well before placing the flowers in it. Conduct this process indoors, with no fans or air blowing near the project. Moist botanicals need to wilt slightly before processing. See "Preparing Botanicals for Tincturing or Infusing" on page 27.

MATERIALS AND EQUIPMENT

Scentless powder, such as arrowroot, tapioca, rice, cornstarch

Fixative, such as powdered orrisroot or powdered ambrette seed

Shallow, closed container

Flowers or leaves

Spatula, large spoon, or piece of stiff cardboard

Chopsticks, tweezers, or slotted spoon

Sieve or stainless steel strainer

Decorative containers for storage

PROCESS

1. Mix the powder of your choice with the powdered fixative.
2. Pour half of the powder into your enfleurage container, and spread it evenly to cover the bottom of the container at least 2 inches (5 cm) deep. A rectangular or square container is best, such as a restaurant steamer tray in a size that suits your project, with a lid that fits snugly. If you're using extremely small flowers or plants, you could use a glass jar or small food storage unit instead.
3. Gently place the properly prepared botanical on the powder base, with edges touching but not overlapping.
4. Pour the remainder of the powder on top of the botanical. Press the powder down very gently to ensure surface contact between the botanical and powder. I use a piece of cardboard or a broad spatula.
5. Loosely cover the container with a lid (but don't tightly seal it), and place it in a warm, dry place, out of the sun.
6. Check the botanical for dryness once a day. You want it to become thoroughly dry, with no moisture remaining. It will typically be dry in one day. When dry, take care not to greatly disturb the powder as you carefully remove the botanical, either by hand or with a pair of tweezers or chopsticks, or a slotted spoon.

(continued)

COLD POWDER ENFLEURAGE (CONT.)

7. Gently tap the botanical with a chopstick as you remove it to release clinging powder. There will always be some powder remaining, but the goal is to shake as much of it as possible into the container.
8. Use the spatula, large spoon, or cardboard to move half the powder to one end of the container, making a mound, but leaving a uniform layer of powder covering the remaining 80 to 90 percent of the bottom of the container's surface area.
9. Recharge the powder with fresh prepared botanical material. Cover the botanical with the powder from the mound.
10. Repeat steps 5 through 9 until the powder is saturated with scent and/or scented to your liking. Use a sieve or strainer to remove any last bits of the botanical from the powder. Place the powder in the decorative container of your choice (see tip below). Make sure to label the container with the type of powder used, botanical name, number of charges, and the date.

TIP: I recommend storing your enfleuraged powders in nonporous containers (such as glass) to help retain their scent. Choose a container with either a perforated shaker top or a removable lid and powder puff. Vintage ones are available on Etsy and other websites. Powder boxes look pretty on a vanity or bureau. These can be modern or vintage, and a fluffy powder puff is delightful to use because it brings a more feminine touch to getting dressed. If you decide to make powder enfleurages to use as deodorants, you may prefer a shaker top container so you just have to shake a little onto your fingers for application.

VAPOR POWDER ENFLEURAGE

After discovering the powder enfleurage information in the book *Natural Perfume*, it occurred to me that I could make vapor essence powder enfleurage with resins, gums, and woods, using an incense warmer. It's easy and fun to do, and you can use the resulting powder as you would other perfumed powders. As in all of my enfleurages, I usually use 1 pound (454 g) of powder per enfleurage, but you can use more or less depending on how much of the botanical you have. As with a simplers' infusion or tincture, you simply keep recharging the powder with fresh botanicals until you've reached the scent you desire, or until the powder seems saturated with scent and can't accept any more.

MATERIALS AND EQUIPMENT

Powder, such as arrowroot, tapioca, rice, cornstarch

Enfleurage vessel large enough to contain the botanical and heat source

Electric incense warmer

Botanical material

Aluminum foil

Glass jar or other nonporous container to store the scented powder

Labels and record-keeping tools

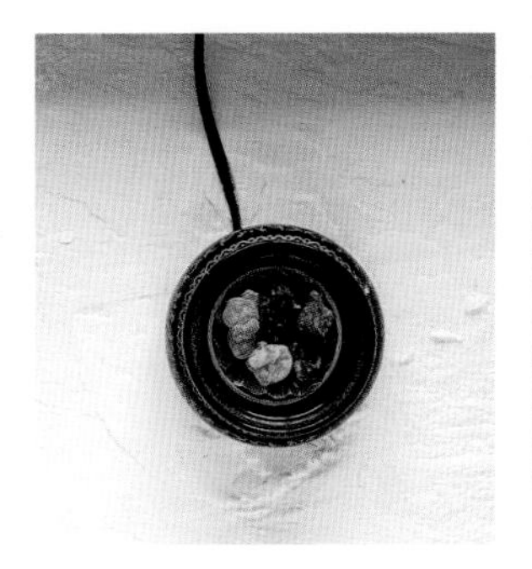

Shown here is an incense warmer containing resins for "hot" powder enfleurage. Have fun experimenting with this easy method.

PROCESS

1. Place the powder inside the enfleurage vessel, at least 2 inches (5 cm) deep.
2. Place the incense warmer into the vessel, on top of the powder.
3. Plug in the warmer and turn it on.
4. Place the botanical onto the heat plate of the warmer.
5. Tightly cover the vessel with aluminum foil, being careful to seal it around the warmer's power cord so that the scent can't escape.
6. Allow the scented vapor to perfume the powder. Recharge the botanical on the warmer's heat plate if you need to make the scent stronger. Do this as many times as necessary to scent the powder to your desired strength. Make sure to keep a record of the number of charges.
7. When the powder is scented to your liking, remove the incense warmer and botanical, and allow the powder to completely cool. Otherwise, it will form condensation, which can cause the powder to clump or cake together, and may attract bacteria.
8. Pour the powder into a clean, airtight, nonporous container for storage. Label the container with the name of the plant, plant part used, type of powder, number of botanical charges, and the date.

TIP: Like the cold-processed enfleurage powders, keep the powder in a glass jar, tightly lidded, or store it in powder shakers. The shakers are inexpensive, and some lovely vintage ones can be found on the Internet or in antique stores. I have some beautiful frosted glass Art Deco containers that I cherish.

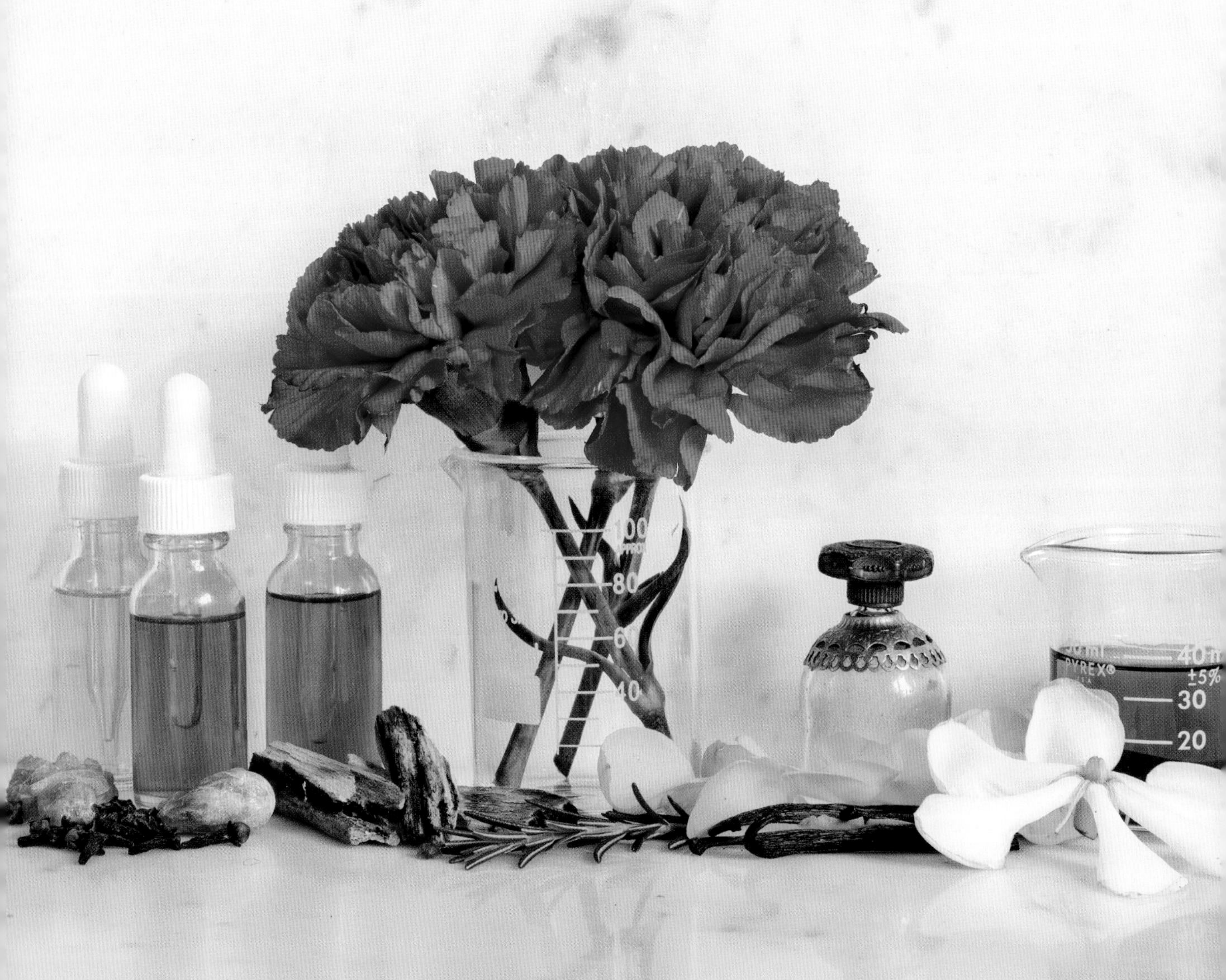
80
40
PYREX®
±5%
30
20

5

PERFUMES FOR BODY, BATH, AND HOME

Now you can begin to really have fun making fragrant products from your extractions and giving gifts to friends and family. The first lovely concoction is perfume, of course! Then we'll see about room, linen, and body sprays, solid perfumes, bath milks, and more. It's so rewarding to make these fragrant products for yourself, as well as for loved ones. Imagine the delight of a little niece receiving a rose-scented solid perfume, or a favorite aunt using a lily of the valley dusting powder. Men will like scented body oil, solid balms, body powders, and colognes.

Left: Shown here from left to right are dropper bottles with tinctures, inspirational flowers about to be extracted for scent, bottles, and beakers with extracts—some of the elements a perfume gardener thinks about and works with when conceptualizing the products and processes.

INTRODUCTION TO PERFUMES

By now, you've probably been spraying on your hydrosols, dabbing your skin with tinctures, pomades, and infusions, playing with all of your extracts, and maybe even mixing them together a little. Next, I want to guide you through blending them into perfumes. You could purchase, or you may already have, some essential oils or absolutes. If you wish, you can use them to enhance or supplement your extracts when you make fragrant products.

Types of Perfume

Most modern natural perfumes contain two types of commercially available aromatic extracts from plants: essential oils and absolutes. For perfume gardeners, this also includes the essential oils, tinctures, pomade extraits, infusions, and other extracts that you make. Using the techniques in this book, you can make several forms of liquid and solid perfume, as follows:

Alcohol based: Worldwide, alcohol-based perfumes are the most popular form of perfume. They are made by dissolving essential oils and absolutes in high-proof alcohol. The alcohol gives them more "lift" and diffusiveness than oil-based perfumes. They can be made for dauber, splash, or spray bottles.

Oil based: Oil perfumes are made by mixing essential oils and absolutes into an oil base, typically jojoba oil or almond oil, which is then allowed to mature until the components blend and marry. Oil perfumes can also be made with oil infusions, either singly (think of a beautiful rose-infused oil) or blended with other oil infusions, or with essential oils and absolutes. The sensuality of anointing skin with a fragrant oil perfume appeals to many people. Oil perfumes are also popular as hair products because they hold the scent for many hours. A small amount rubbed between your palms and smoothed over your hair makes a scented hair conditioner that provides extra shine.

Water based: Water-based perfumes, such as rose water and orange flower water, have a long history in perfumery. By now you know about hydrosols, also known as floral waters, hydrolats, or distillate waters. They are the water product that results from the distillation process that yields essential oils. Hydrosols are gaining in popularity in perfumery because of their usefulness in skin care and home fragrance products. They can be used as single scents, or blended to create a perfume with complexity.

Solid: Solid perfumes are scented balms made with melted beeswax (or other natural waxes) and butters or oils, and fragranced with essential oils and absolutes. The same oil extractions that are used for oil perfumes can be used in combination with beeswax, other solid waxes, or nut butters to make solid perfumes. These perfumes are typically poured into small metal cases, such as pillboxes or decorative watchcases or beautiful compacts, or even into jewelry pieces, such as lockets, and allowed to harden. Their portability in a purse or pocket makes them popular.

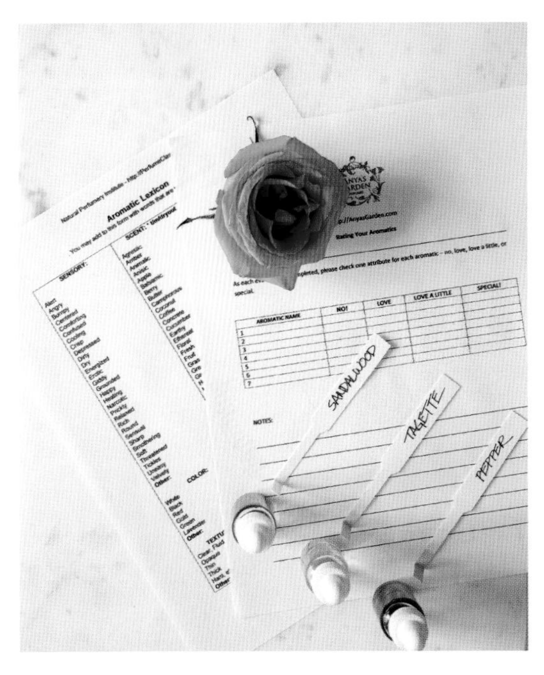

Using Scents Safely with Scent Strips

You may be tempted to use essential oils or absolutes directly on your skin, but please don't. They are so concentrated that they can cause irritation or a rash. Worst of all, they can cause long-term sensitization so that you may not be able to use a particular oil ever again without having a reaction. It's possible that you might subsequently have a reaction to other oils in the same family.

It is important that you use scent strips to test your perfumes while you're blending them to reduce skin contact until they're properly diluted. Additionally, before you begin blending alcohol perfumes, review "Safety Considerations," beginning on page 23.

Scent strips provide a quick and inexpensive way to test and evaluate aromatics. You can use them to sample single aromatics, such as when categorizing your aromatics. You can also use several scent strips to evaluate multiple aromatics at the same time, such as determining which aromatics blend well together when you're building a perfume.

This is where note taking is absolutely necessary. Don't depend on your memory. Making perfumes requires a lot of note taking, especially if you wish to duplicate a perfume in the future. If you don't take notes, or if you lose them, I predict you'll be heartbroken. I write down my notes on paper as I evaluate, then type them up and store them on paper, online, and on my hard drive. I suggest you do the same, so you can have them available whenever you need them.

Include in your notes a rating—as in the following table—for your like or dislike of the aromatic, as well as your impression of how the aromatic smells to you and makes you feel.

Strongly Dislike	Dislike	Neutral	Like a Lot	Love
1	2	3	4	5

To help you develop the scent vocabulary to use with your aromatics, use the following:

AROMATIC LEXICON TABLE					
Sensory	**Scent: Top, middle, drydown**		**Place memory**	**Color**	**Texture/ Visual**
Alert	Amber	Metallic	Bed	White	Clear
Angry	Apple	Milky	Church	Black	Fluid
Bumpy	Balsamic	Minty	City	Red	Opaque
Centered	Berry	Musky	Family	Gold	Thin
Comforting	Burnt	Peppery	Forest	Green	Thick
Confused	Buttery	Piney	Friends	Lavender	Hard
Cooling	Camphorous	Powdery	Holiday		
Crisp	Caramel	Pungent	Job		
Depressed	Citrusy	Resinous	Laundry		
Dirty	Clove	Rosy	Lover		
Dry	Coconut	Sharp	Mall		
Energized	Coffee	Skunky	Mountain		
Erotic	Concrete	Smoky	Ocean		
Ethereal	Cucumber	Soapy	Park		
Giddy	Earthy	Sour	Person		
Grounded	Farm	Spicy	Picnic		
Happy	Floral	Sulfurous	Restaurant		
Heating	Fresh	Sweet	Seashore		
Narcotic	Fruity	Tar	Section of city		
Prickly	Grassy	Tea			
Relaxed	Greasy	Toasted			
Rich	Hairy	Tropical			
Round	Herbal	Urinous			
Sensual	Honey	Vanilla			
Sharp	Leather	Waxy			
Smothering	Licorice	Wine			
Soft	Marine	Woody			
Ticklish	Meadow				
Uneasy					
Velvety					

CONSTRUCTING A SCENT

In this section, you will learn how to categorize and evaluate all of your aromatics so that you can determine which ones work well with one another, and how to blend them to make your own custom scents.

All botanical scents are classified as top, middle, or base notes, based on evaporation and longevity, defined by how long the scent lasts on skin, or on a paper scent strip, until you can no longer smell it.

- Top notes last from two to twenty minutes.
- Middle notes last from two to eight hours.
- Base notes last up to twenty-four hours.

For example, a tincture, infusion, or essential oil of an aromatic top note, such as juniper berry, can disappear within twenty minutes of application. Middle notes, such as rose, bay leaf, jasmine, and rosemary, are more long lasting, providing the "heart" of a perfume, for two to eight hours—sometimes longer. The longest-lasting scents are base note aromatics, such as patchouli or ambrette seed. Base notes are the anchors of perfumery, often lasting up to twenty-four hours or more.

Essential oils, hydrosols, and absolutes that you distill can fall into any of the top, middle, or base note categories, depending on their source material. Tinctures, infusions, and enfleurage products may not last as long as their essential oil or absolute counterparts because they are not as concentrated. Also, because body heat accelerates a scent's evaporation, scents can evaporate more quickly from your skin than they do from a scent strip.

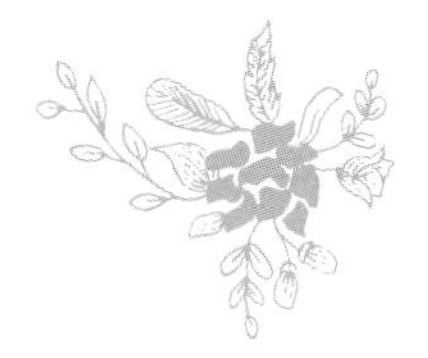

Here is the standard process for categorizing aromatics in the perfume industry.

It isn't necessary to inhale deeply, or to smell the aromatic at great length—you only need a little time with a scent to perceive its characteristics.

1. Write down the name of the aromatic and the type (e.g., essential oil, hydrosol) on one end of the scent strip.
2. Dip the very tip of the scent strip into the aromatic, wetting ⅛ to ¼ inch (3 to 6 mm) of it.
3. Holding the scent strip perpendicular to your nose, at about 1 inch (2.5 cm) below it, waft the aromatic by gently moving the strip back and forth while softly breathing in the aromatic.
4. Write your impression of the aromatic, using the table on page 102.
5. Revisit smelling the scent strip twenty minutes later. If the scent has faded considerably, it is a top note.
6. Revisit smelling the scent strip two hours later. If it has faded only a bit, it is a middle note.
7. Revisit smelling the scent strip five hours later. If the scent is still strong, it is a base note.
8. Repeat steps 1 through 7 with subsequent aromatics that you're evaluating for your perfume.
9. Write down your observations for each aromatic, grouped by top, middle, and base categories.

Planning Your Scent Blend and Evaluating the Aromatics

In order to create pleasing scents, it's necessary for you to plan how your product will smell and perform. You need to continue evaluating your aromatics and to compare them with one another. It may seem exciting to blend together everything you have extracted, but without planning and evaluation, you'll likely end up with a muddied mess, with no specific scent or any defining note, and the blend will smell dense and uninteresting, or the aromas will clash.

When you're planning your perfume, the first step is deciding on an aromatic group so that your perfume has a theme. What type of perfume do you like? Floral? Spicy? Green?

Study the following aromatic groups to see how your extracts fit into them, then choose the group(s) that you want to define your perfume.

Some aromatics fit into more than one group. For example, patchouli is both earthy and woody. Lavender is both floral and herbal. If you have essences that are not listed here, look at the list for ones that are similar to help you decide which aromatic groups your extracts belong to.

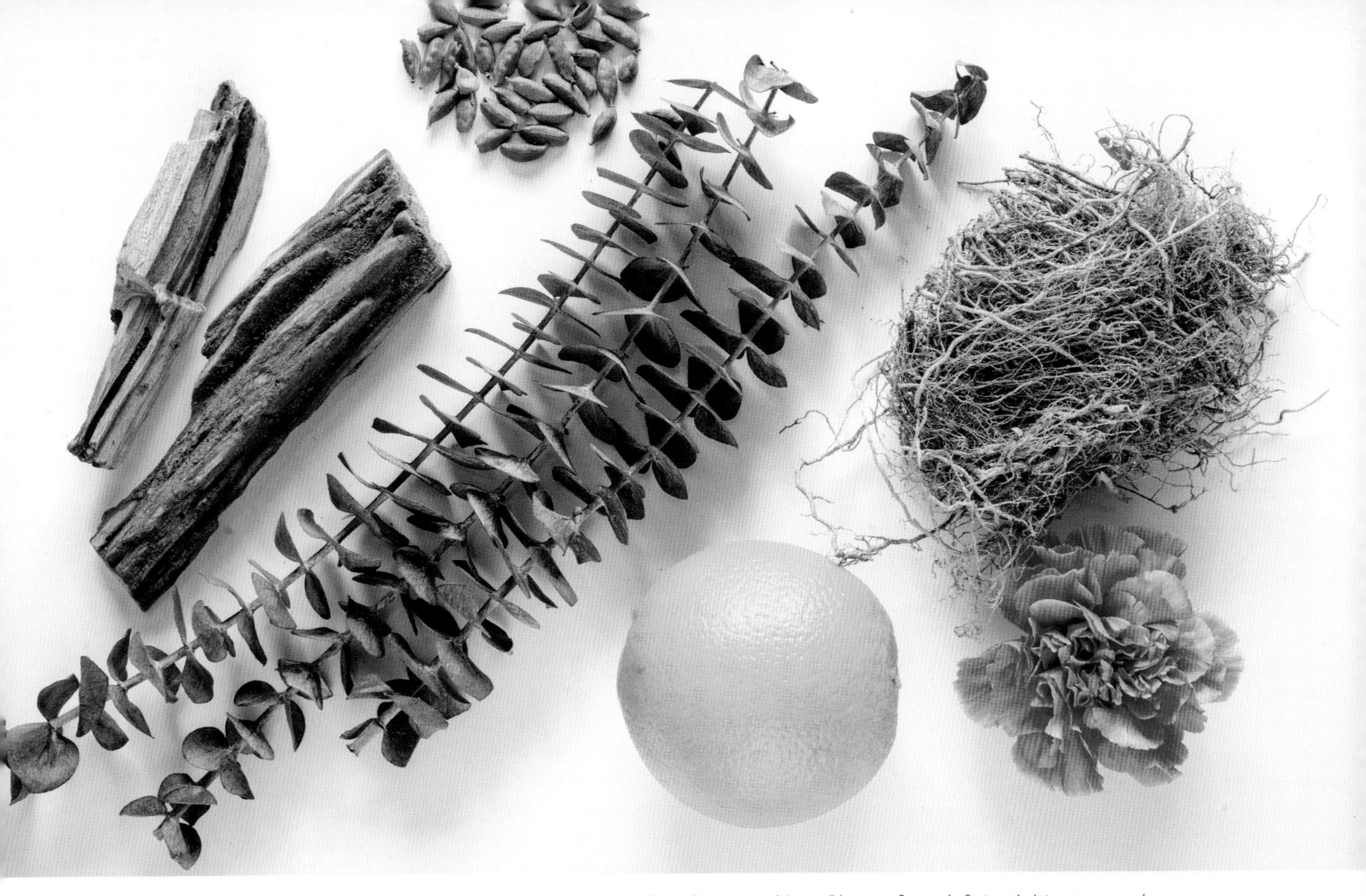

Learning about aromatic groups is a basic component of perfume making. Shown from left to right are woody (palo santo), green (eucalyptus), spicy (cardamom seeds), citrusy (orange), earthy (vetiver), and floral (carnation).

Citrusy: Sweet orange, pink grapefruit, lemongrass

Earthy: Oakmoss, patchouli, vetiver

Floral: Jasmine, rose, ylang-ylang, lavender, neroli, hyacinth

Fruity: Besides actual fruits, includes fruity flowers such as chamomile and osmanthus

Green: Clary sage, violet leaf, spearmint, peppermint

Herbal: Juniper berry, basil, clary sage, lavender, rosemary

Spicy: Cardamom, cinnamon, coriander, nutmeg

Woody: Cedar, pine, patchouli, sandalwood

After you choose a theme—for example, citrusy—you can modify it with some enhancers. Perhaps a touch of florals, some coriander or juniper for the top, and some woods for the base to complement the citrus essences.

Focusing Your Theme: Fragrance Family

The next step in planning your perfume is to select a fragrance family, which helps you focus your perfume's theme. In the late 1800s, perfume companies developed fragrance families as marketing guides for the customer, giving a good description of the main components and the main theme of the perfume. They usually contain a combination of aromatic groups. The following examples are only some of the combinations that you might consider for your fragrance family.

Citrus	Floral	Woody
	Single floral	Woody (general)
Citrus (general)	Floral bouquet	Conifer citrus woody
Spicy citrus	Green floral	Spicy woody
Woody citrus	Woody fruity floral	Amber woody
Floral woody citrus	Woody floral	Spicy leathery woody
	Fruity floral	Fruity woody

There are many other fragrance family combinations; you can be creative and make up your own, if you wish. You can also search the Internet for more fragrance family examples.

Evaluating Aromatics

After choosing an aromatic group and fragrance family for your perfume, you need to evaluate the aromatics in the group you chose. First, decide what smells good together. Some aromatics smell beautiful separately but clash fiercely when combined.

With a scent strip holder or other apparatus of your choice, find a way to hold several scent strips you're evaluating, while keeping them separated so that they don't touch one another. If you don't have a holder, you can bend the scent strip in the middle and place the flat, nonaromatic side down on an impervious surface, so that the end with the aromatic is facing upward. See example on page 101.

Gather the aromatics of your choice—the ones that smell best to you, or that are calling to you in the moment—and follow these simple steps to evaluate the scent.

1. Use a scent strip to sample aromatic number 1 of your choice—for example gardenia—so you can become acquainted with all of the nuances of the oil.
2. Dip a new scent strip into a second aromatic, such as ylang-ylang, and study it.
3. Redip each scent strip into its original aromatic and, holding them side-by-side, smell them together. Do you like the combination? Maybe not.
4. Make notes, and use your observations to help you build your perfume.

TIP: Do not store your unused scent strips near your aromatics. They can absorb the scents that escape into the air from the bottles, even when the bottles are tightly closed. You may wish to store them in a glass jar with a tight-fitting lid.

BLENDING SCENTS IN LIQUID PERFUME

When you're blending scents, you want a harmonious combination. The well-blended finished product consists of:

- The flighty top notes often provide a zesty or spicy introduction to the perfume. Think citrus, coriander seed, or juniper berry.
- The heart notes of the perfume, after the top notes waft away, are often a floral blend, such as rose, lily, jasmine, and similar oils, providing a lovely interlude of pretty and interesting fragrance. This phase is often what people look for, and want, as the identifying theme of a perfume.
- The robust base notes, such as patchouli, labdanum, and vetiver, are the final, sensual, soft remnants of the perfume, often providing delight as we awaken the morning after having worn the perfume, providing a gentle memory of the perfume.

For the hobbyist perfumer, quick estimates are acceptable when you begin blending. More experienced perfumers will follow very precise amounts because they need to know the exact proportions and how to replicate the scent for sale, but you don't need to be exact to have some fun with your perfume. Follow these basic proportions, then adjust them to your liking as you develop a perfume:

- **Top:** 20 percent
- **Middle:** 50 percent
- **Base:** 30 percent

A lot of recommended percentages in perfumery books are much lower for middle notes and much higher for base notes—often the reverse of what I recommend. I've discovered over years of making perfume that because so many of the middle notes have a decent longevity of three to five hours, combining them with a lower ratio of base notes creates a more than adequate longevity for the perfume. In addition, we have so many more middle notes to choose from, in comparison to the number of base notes available, so you have a great variety of aromatics to work with.

NOTE: If you're making an oil or solid perfume, you may want to increase the top notes to 30 percent, and reduce the base notes to 20 percent, because oils or fats dampen the top notes, and oil and wax slow the perfume's evaporation from skin; they assist the base notes in making the perfume last longer on skin.

Try your hand at blending tiny amounts to see what you like. You will be excited and want to mix your beloved blend immediately into the diluent alcohol or oil to finish the perfume, but wait! Put an identical blend aside and allow it to mature for several weeks to several months, and you may find it has evolved into something a lot more beautiful, or perhaps not so wonderful. This is the mystery and adventure in perfume making, and you will experience it.

After you have made some test perfumes using tiny amounts of aromatics to conserve them, you can graduate to making 5 milliliter perfumes, and this is the amount we'll use in our liquid perfume recipe on page 113. Start small. You can always increase the size of your perfumes, but while you're still learning and experimenting, small is best. You can make more types of perfumes, and get a lot of feedback from others on the blends. Just think how boring life would be if everyone liked and wore the same kind of perfume. One ounce (28 ml) of perfume might seems like a small amount, but it might take months to use it up, and variety and understanding how the aromatics interact is the goal for the perfume gardener.

Once you mix your blend into alcohol to create a perfume, this is when it really gets exciting, as you will see how the alcohol "opens up" the aromatics. It reveals their inner beauty and also helps make them diffuse more in the air.

On average, keep in mind that 1 milliliter of essential oils, extraits, tinctures, or absolutes contains about 20 drops. This may vary if you have a particularly thick aromatic, so use your judgment when counting your drops. Use a standard dropper so that your measurements are consistent.

Percentage Guide for Perfume Types

No matter whether you plan to use alcohol or oil as a base for your perfume, the following table gives percentage ranges for the essential oils and diluents that are used for perfumes, from pure perfume to a light eau de cologne, or "splash" fragrance.

NOTE: There is only one type of oil perfume; it doesn't occur as eau de parfum, eau de toilette, eau de cologne, or splash. Also, never add any ingredients that contain water to an oil perfume.

Type of Perfume	% of Essential Oil or Extraits	% of Diluent: Alcohol/Oil/Tincture*
Perfume	20–30	70–80
Eau de parfum	15–20	80–85
Eau de toilette	10–15	85–90
Eau de cologne	5–10	90–95
Splash	2–5	95–98

* Instead of using pure alcohol as a diluent, you may wish to use 100 percent tincture, or you can use part tincture and part alcohol.

For alcohol or oil perfumes, I recommend limiting the maximum concentration of essential oil to 30 percent. For example, if you have 30 milliliters of essential oil, dilute it with 70 milliliters of alcohol to make 100 milliliters of perfume.

For brevity, the word perfume in this book can mean perfume, eau de parfum, eau de toilette, cologne, or splash. You decide which strength of perfume to make, and then follow the general instructions on dilution percentages for that.

Remember that the easiest way to measure liquids for your perfumes and scented products is by volume. You will need to have small-scale volumetric beakers and graduated cylinders to accurately measure the precise concentrations (see page 17 for the types I recommend).

CHECKLIST BEFORE MAKING LIQUID PERFUME

The following is a quick checklist that briefly touches on all of the planning steps to take before you begin blending your perfume.

1. Determine the aromatic group(s) you like the best, and then determine the fragrance family you want to create from a blend of two or more aromatic groups. Alternatively, instead of focusing on a fragrance family, you could opt to experiment with just one or two aromatic groups.

2. Gather the tinctures (alcohol-based perfume), infusions (oil-based perfume), enfleurage extraits you've made, and any purchased oils and absolutes you may need as supplements to your own extracts in order to achieve your desired fragrance family type.

3. Systematically experiment with all of the aromatics by using scent strips to find the combination that is most pleasing to you, and write down your findings as the basis for your perfume.

4. Determine what aromatics percentages to use in your perfume by referring to the recommended top, middle, and base note proportions on page 107, recognizing that alcohol perfumes may require slightly different ratios than oil perfumes.

5. Determine the amount of perfume you will make.

6. Using the table in "Percentage Guide for Perfume Types" on page 108, calculate the amounts of diluent and aromatics that you need.

7. Assemble the equipment listed in the next section on a surface that will not be marred by any spills, or put down a protective cover; both the aromatics and alcohol can damage most surfaces because they are solvents.

8. Keep good written or typed notes on the outcome for all of your work. I also scan the notes and save them online in the cloud.

IMPORTANT MATERIALS AND EQUIPMENT NEEDED TO MAKE LIQUID PERFUMES

Here is a basic list of all the supplies you will need in the perfume recipes on the following pages.

- Base liquid of your choice—190-proof alcohol, carrier oil, scented oil, or tincture that can replace all or a portion of the alcohol in the perfume
- Scented extracts—garden extract oils that you made and/or essential oils or absolutes that you purchased (optional)
- Water or hydrosol
- Beakers—10-milliliter, 50-milliliter, and larger-capacity beakers if you're making more than 1 ounce (28 ml)
- Graduated cylinders—from 10 milliliter to 100 milliliter
- Glass or stainless steel funnel to easily pour your finished perfume into a decorative bottle
- Glass droppers with Monprene bulbs in a standard size
- Stainless steel measuring spoons (optional)
- Scent strips
- Bottle(s) for the finished perfume
- Label(s) for the finished perfume

REMINDER: If you plan to make an alcohol-based perfume, you need 190-proof alcohol. If you can get only lower-proof alcohol, you can use it, but your perfume will look cloudy. The oils will likely separate and float on the top, so you'll need to shake the finished perfume each time before use to disperse the aromatics in the alcohol. This will not affect the quality of the perfume—it's merely cosmetic. Opaque bottles are best for cloudy perfumes, to hide the cloudiness.

If you plan to make oil-based perfume, jojoba and moringa oils are typically used.

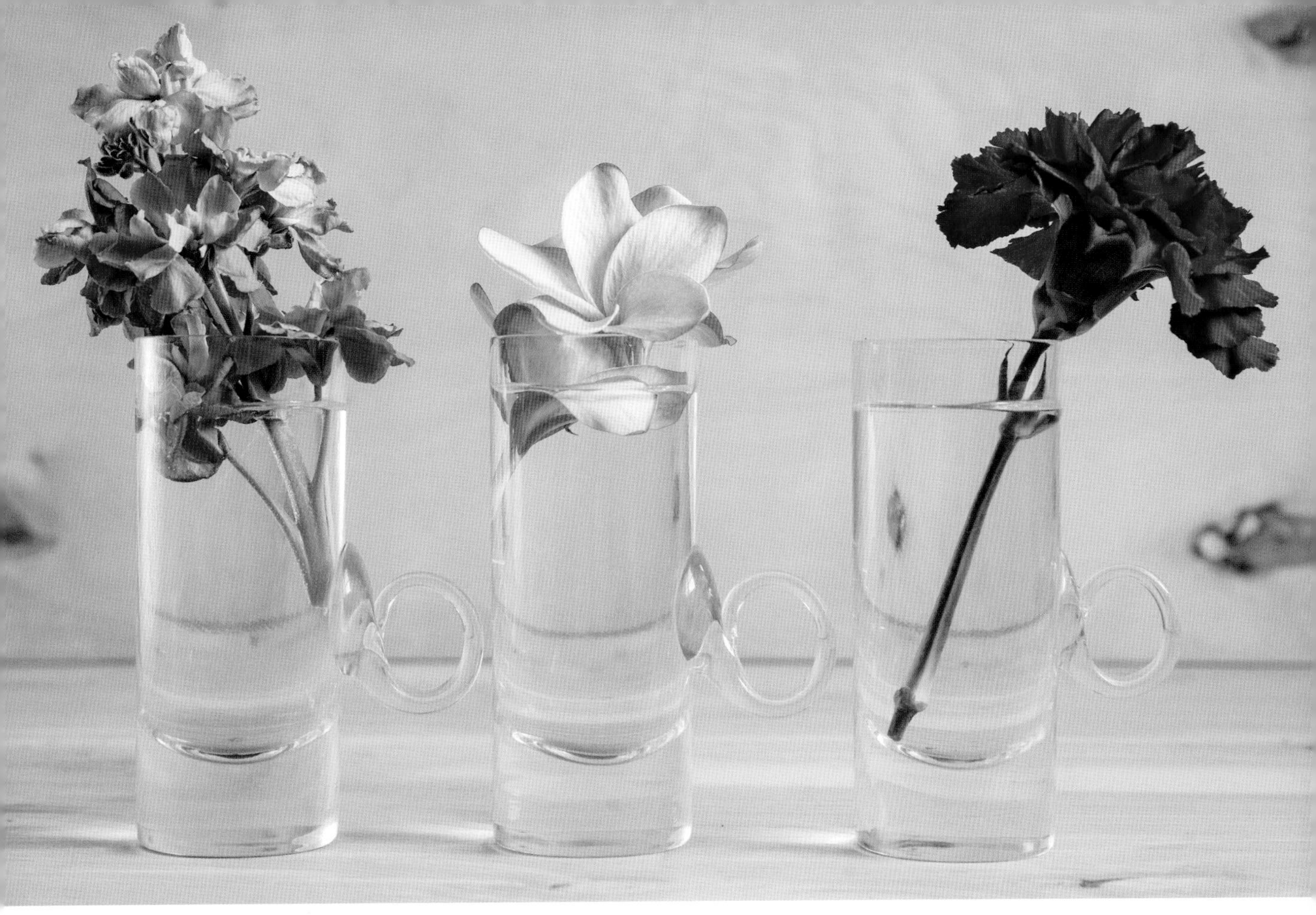

For those in cooler climates, night-scented stock (left) is lovely and easy to grow. Frangipani, or plumeria (middle), has an intoxicating, sophisticated fragrance. And who doesn't love carnation (right)? Not the scentless carnations from stores, but the fresh, bright, clove-like carnation.

FINAL NOTE BEFORE MAKING PERFUMED PROJECTS

In the next section, I give you my tried-and-true formulas for products for your body and home. This is where all of your hard work pays off and you learn to use the fragrant extraits that you made!

Each reader will have his or her own unique array of homemade extracts and purchased essential oils and absolutes to play with while creating these products. The recipes I'm sharing are meant to be tailored to your fragrant supplies on hand. You may not have ylang-ylang tincture, but you may have ylang-ylang oil. The guidelines for the aromatics in the blends are just that. Don't forget to use scent strips to evaluate how the proposed recipes appeal to you, and feel free to alter the ingredients as your nose guides you.

Use the proportions and measurements for the water/hydrosol or tincture-based sprays interchangeably! If you like a recipe for a tincture spray because the ingredients appeal to you, but you want it in the form of a water/hydrosol spray, just use the water/hydrosol proportions for your ingredients.

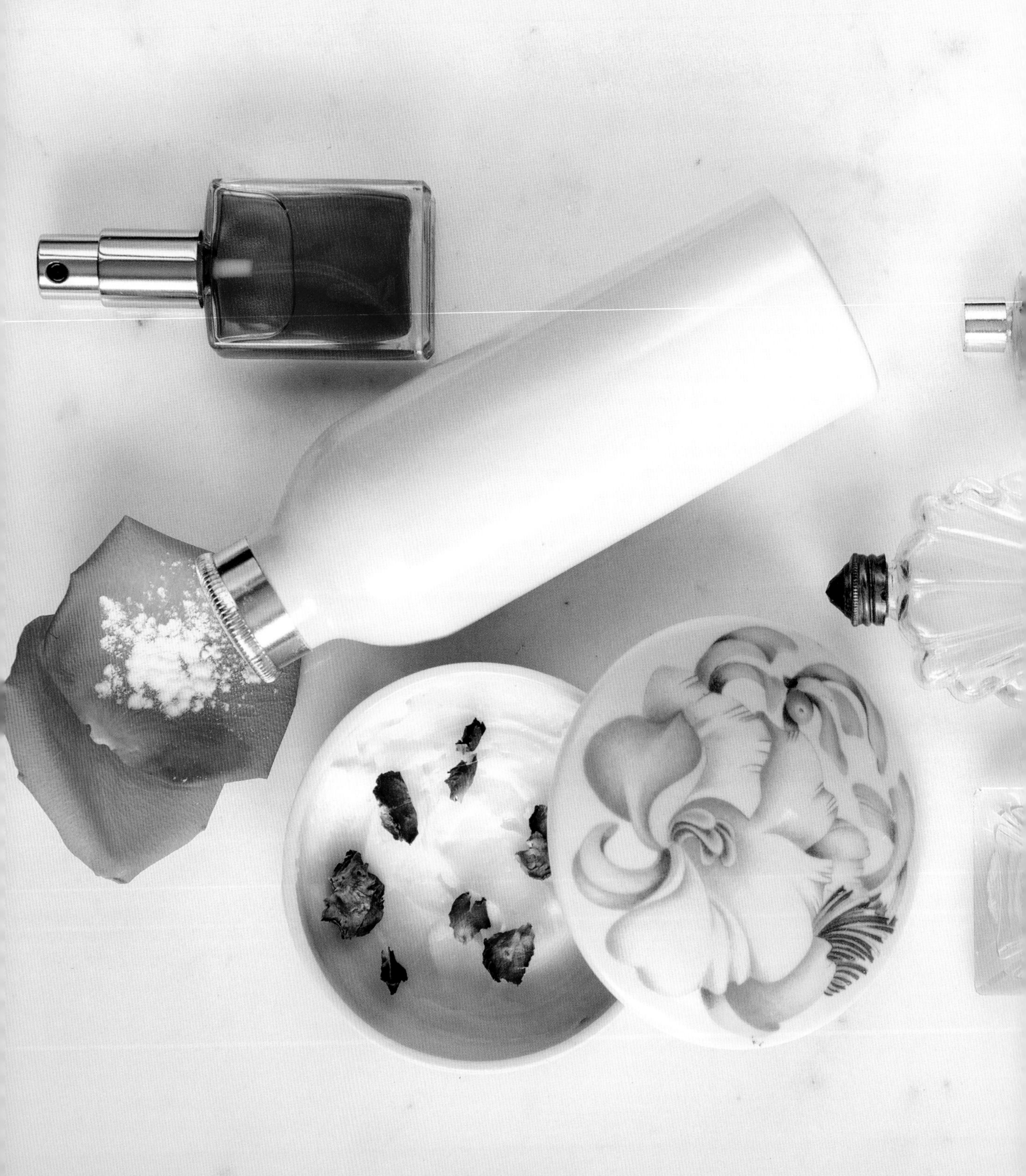

LIQUID PERFUME

Whether you are creating an alcohol perfume or an oil perfume, instructions for creating it are the same; the only difference is that oil perfumes typically need a higher percentage of top notes because the oil dampens them.

This starter recipe produces one 5-milliliter perfume. I always recommend making small batches of perfume. This helps to conserve your essences, because you'll likely need to make some adjustments in various aromatic amounts during the blending process. Also worth noting, after blending and diluting, you'll need to allow the perfume to mature for several weeks to several months to allow the scents to marry.

After the basic recipe, you will find three sample recipes of aromatic blends that I particularly love. These are meant to be a guide; use them to evaluate the scented products you have made and compare similar stock you have on hand. Instead of 190-proof alcohol, you may wish to use a lightly-scented tincture or infusion as the diluent. After all, it's made with 190-proof alcohol, and perhaps you didn't have enough recharges to make a strongly-scented tincture or infusion, but you love the light scent, and you can incorporate it as the diluent. Play around, and have fun!

MATERIALS AND EQUIPMENT

4 ml diluent—190-proof alcohol or oil

1 ml total of aromatic(s)—such as essential oils, tinctures, extraits, and infusions

Dropper

Blending vessel—such as a beaker, a graduated cylinder, or other nonreactive vessel with a spout

Glass or stainless steel stirring rod

Distilled water or hydrosol (optional)

Label and recordkeeping tools

Funnel

Small vial or bottle

Decorative bottles for finished perfume

PROCESS

1. Decide what type of perfume you want to make. For perfumes that are meant to be for massage or body perfume, oil is the diluent of choice. If you want a more classic, uplifting type of perfume that can be dispersed through the air, use alcohol.
2. Choose which aromatics you wish to blend based on the top/middle/base note percentages. You can refer to the plant profiles in Chapter 6 if needed, where each plant's profile says whether it is a top, middle, or base note.
3. Use the chart below for the specific number of drops per aromatic. Make sure to use a standard dropper for consistency.

Blending Percentage	Number of Drops
20% top note(s)	4 drops
50% middle note(s)	10 drops
30% base note(s)	6 drops
Total	20 drops / 1 ml

(continued)

LIQUID PERFUME (CONT.)

4. Blend your aromatics in the blending vessel with the stirring rod. Use a graduated beaker or small beaker with markings showing milliliter volume in 1-milliliter increments. I prefer a 10-milliliter graduated beaker for this. You should have 1 milliliter total. Make sure to keep written notes on the amounts of each aromatic.
5. Dilute your final blend with 4 milliliters of alcohol or oil. This will make a classic perfume. If you'd like to make a eau de parfum, eau de toilette, eau de cologne, or splash, refer to page 108 for the proper proportions to adjust.
6. For alcohol-based perfumes only, you can add a small amount of distilled water or hydrosol to the perfume. This can help diffuse the perfume and softens the effect of the alcohol on your skin, and can also help to slow evaporation. Add the water in tiny amounts—even as little as several drops at a time—to your blend, stirring gently with a glass or stainless steel rod after each addition. If you add too much water, your blend will become cloudy. Refrigerate overnight to see if the cloudiness clears.
7. Pour the diluted blend into an airtight container and close it tightly. Label the container with the aromatics used, the amounts of each, the type of diluent, and the date. Allow the blend to mature in a cool, dry place for several weeks to several months. This is an important step, as without proper aging, a blend might smell beautiful at first, only to become unacceptable over time. Conversely, a blend that smells rough at first might mellow and marry into something rich and beautiful when given time to age properly.
8. When you determine the perfume is perfectly scented and aged, pour the finished perfume into pretty bottles for use.

FOREST

4 drops linden (top note)

10 drops conifer (middle note)

6 drops vetiver (base note)

MORNING SUN

4 drops grapefruit (top note)

10 drops jasmine (middle note)

6 drops vanilla (base note)

GARDEN OF EDEN

4 drops lavender (top note)

10 drops ylang-ylang (middle note)

6 drops frankincense (base note)

TIP: To increase the amount of perfume you make, keep the ratios the same as you scale up the recipe. For example, to make a 10-milliliter perfume, use 8 milliliters of diluent and 8 drops of top note(s), 20 drops of middle note(s), and 12 drops of base note(s) for a total of 40 drops of aromatics.

SOLID PERFUME

Solid perfumes are fun to make and easy to carry with you in a bag or pocket. With a tight-fitting lid or a screw top, they're pretty impervious to leaking, breaking, or opening and ruining your bag, and they're very handy. Many people delight in the aesthetics of pouring the hot, molten perfume and beeswax mixture into a decorative tin or porcelain case and allowing it to solidify. The many uses include softening your hands and working a little into your hair for fragrant moisturizing. Unlike liquid alcohol perfumes, the top notes are often dampened by the modern solid perfume process, so you'll want to test adding top notes in excess of your original formula.

NOTE: I like to make my solid perfume a bit harder than normal because I live in the tropics, and the hot weather can soften or melt it. The recipe uses the formula that I need for my climate. I recommend adjusting the amounts to your own climate. Also, this recipe makes a small 6-milliliter batch of solid perfume. This is a good amount for a test on scent and degree of hardness. Feel free to double or triple the recipe as you'd like.

MATERIALS AND EQUIPMENT

¾–1 tsp (3.5–5 g) beeswax granules or pastilles (based on your climate)

Small double boiler (or use a small heat-resistant bowl and hotplate)

5 ml fixed oil or carrier oil—such as light olive, almond, grapeseed, jojoba, moringa, or scented oil

30 drops of essential oil or absolute oil

Toothpicks or skewers to stir the melted perfume

Small containers for the finished perfume

PROCESS

1. Begin melting the beeswax in a double boiler over boiling water. You may also use a hot plate and a heat-resistant bowl, called a "crucible." It will take a couple of minutes for the granules to melt completely.
2. Remove the double boiler or crucible from the heat for just a few seconds and add the oil and essential oils to the melted wax. Instead of using a plain carrier oil, this also could be an infused perfume oil you've made. Use a toothpick or skewer to stir the wax, oil, and essential oils together.
3. Return the double boiler to the boiling water (or the crucible to the hot plate) for about 5 seconds, constantly stirring the contents to mix and melt. Promptly remove it from the heat to avoid dampening the scent of your perfume.
4. Immediately pour the hot perfume into your chosen vessel and let it cool on a flat surface for about 15 minutes, or until firm. Voilà! Your solid perfume is ready to use.

TIP: For easy cleanup, it's best to remove as much of the solid perfume from the vessel you heated it in as soon as possible because the beeswax will harden quickly. If you can't clean it immediately, that's okay. Gently heat the bowl or pan again, and wipe it with a paper towel, making sure to get all of the wax and perfume residue. Then wash it in hot, soapy water.

EASY POMADE SEMI-SOLID PERFUME METHOD

Don't feel like going through all the melting and mixing of traditional solid perfume? If you have some pomade you've made, just follow these easy instructions as an alternative to traditional solid perfume. The resulting product has the consistency of whipped butter rather than a solid perfume cake.

MATERIALS AND EQUIPMENT

Small pretty container

Scented pomade

Essential oil(s), infused oil(s), and/or absolute oil(s)

Toothpick or skewer

Label and recordkeeping tools

PROCESS

1. Find a pleasing little screw-top container for your perfume, and pack it about half full of the pomade.
2. Using a blend that you like from the process in "Evaluating Aromatics" (page 106), gather your chosen essential oils, absolutes, and infused oils. Tinctures are not used in solid perfumes. Blend the oils in even ratios of 1:1:1. For example, ten drops of each.
3. Use a toothpick or skewer to mix the oils into the pomade.
4. Slowly add the rest of the pomade, continuing to stir until all are blended.
5. Close the container, label it, and enjoy your quickie whipped butter-style perfume!

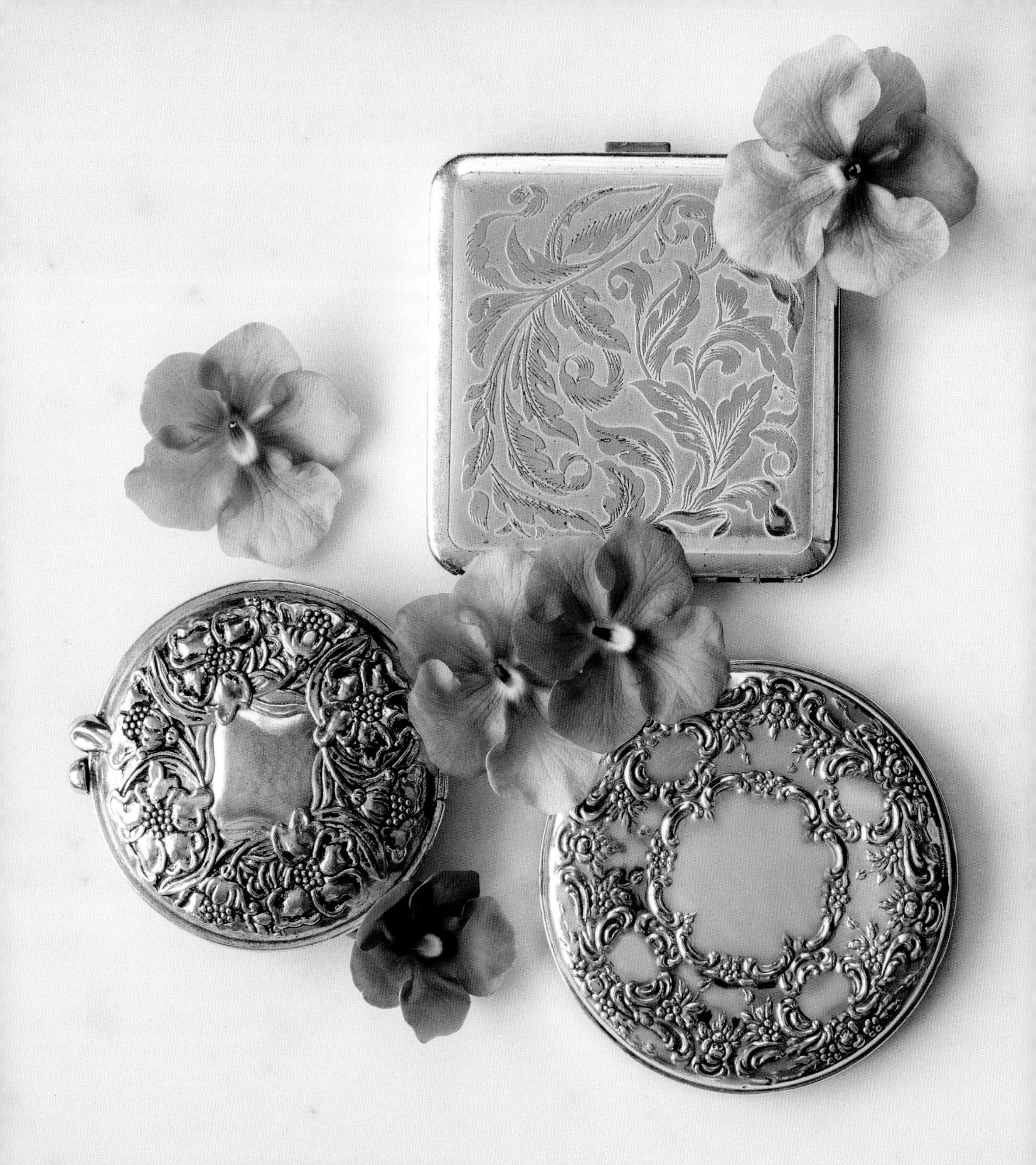

BODY SPRAY/WATER PERFUME

The main ingredient of body spray is water. Because of this, body sprays are often called water perfumes. Their scent comes from essential oils and/or hydrosols. Most water perfumes can be sprayed on fabric without staining, but always test first in an inconspicuous place, such as an inside seam or hem. To more closely control your final fragrance, follow the aromatic group/fragrance family instructions for liquid perfumes (page 106).

You need to add enough 190-proof ethanol to protect the distilled water or hydrosol from microbial growth, and to help the mixture of essential oils and water dissolve into the solution. I use 20 percent 190-proof alcohol for this purpose. You can scale the measurements up or down, depending on the size of spray you wish to make. For each project, your percentages will be 75 percent distilled water or hydrosol, 20 percent alcohol, and 5 percent essential oils or absolutes. The main recipe is a basic formula that you can customize however you'd like. It yields 8 ounces (approximately 236 ml). I've also provided a few of my favorite recipes for you to try out.

MATERIALS AND EQUIPMENT

Graduated beaker to hold 8 oz (236 ml)

Glass or stainless steel stirring rod or stainless steel skewer

8-oz (236-ml) spray bottle

12 ml essential oils or absolutes (5 percent)

47 ml 190-proof alcohol (20 percent)

177 ml distilled water or hydrosol (75 percent)

Label and recordkeeping tools

PROCESS

1. Sterilize the beaker, stirring rod or skewer, spray bottle, and spray top before adding any liquids (see "Safely Cleaning Equipment for Projects" on page 21, if needed).
2. Add the essential oils and/or absolutes and the alcohol to the beaker. Stir with the rod or skewer to blend, cover to prevent evaporation, then allow them to further blend for about 30 minutes.
3. Write down your formula.
4. After the half hour, blend the mixture with the distilled water or hydrosol. Pour the solution into your sterilized spray bottle.
5. Screw on the spray top, label the bottle, and your perfume is ready to use! If you added essential oils or absolutes, you may need to shake the bottle each time before spraying because they will not dissolve completely. You can choose an opaque bottle if you don't want to see the separate layers of the oil and waters.

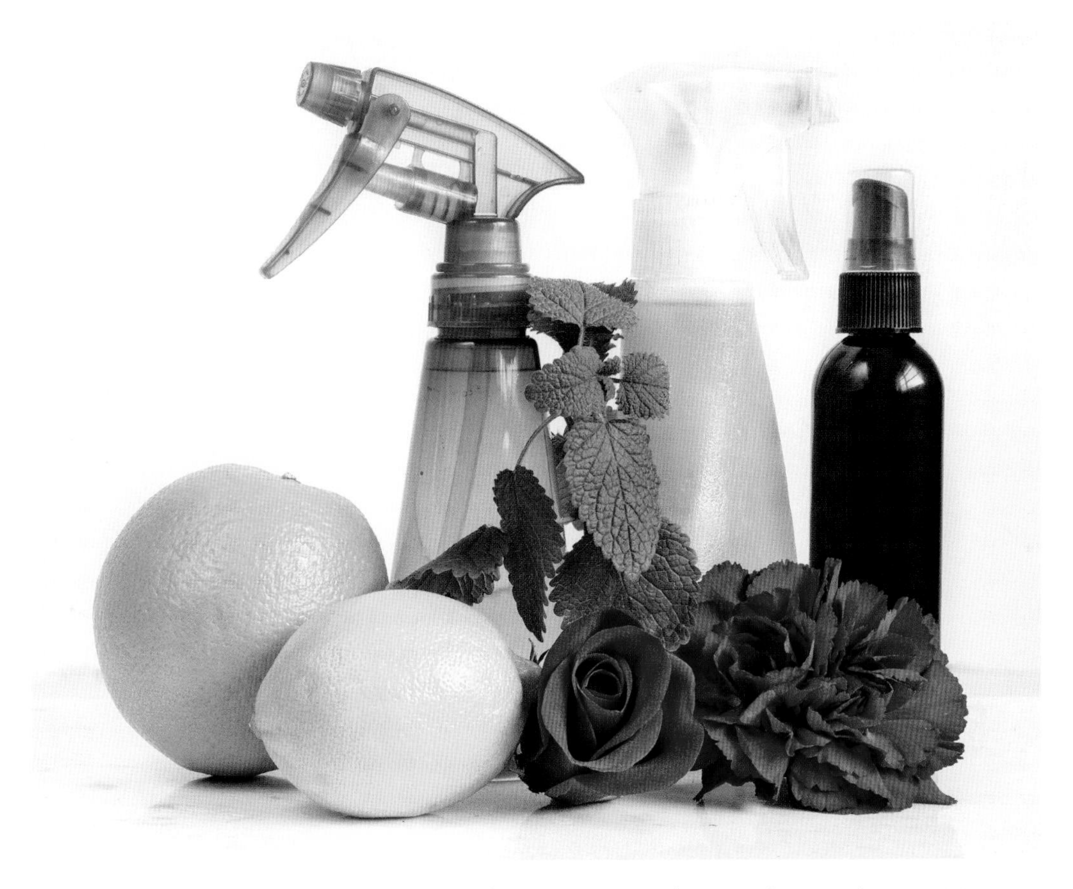

A light, delightful water perfume is perfect for hot, summer days, or when you just want to gently mist your body or hair with a subtle scent. Spray bottles can be kept in the refrigerator for an extra cooling effect.

Floral Spicy Water Perfume

4 ml rose or rose geranium essential oil

4 ml coriander seed essential oil

4 ml lavender essential oil

47 ml 190-proof alcohol

177 ml distilled water or hydrosol (patchouli hydrosol or a light, woody-scented hydrosol would be a supportive base for this blend)

Refreshing Water Perfume

4 ml spearmint or other mint essential oil, or peppermint for a really cooling effect

4 ml lemongrass essential oil

4 ml eucalyptus essential oil

47 ml 190-proof alcohol

177 ml distilled water or hydrosol (rosemary hydrosol, or one of the mints, would add a lot of freshness to this blend)

ROOM AND LINEN SPRAYS

Tinctures and hydrosols, or tinctures blended with hydrosols and perhaps a touch of essential oils or absolutes, are beautiful additions to your household fragrance products. You can make a different scented spray for each room of your home, or for holiday themes. Nothing could be easier or more rewarding, and you'll love that you have truly captured perfume from your garden and made nontoxic, 100 percent natural fragrance sprays for you and your family.

There is no need to add any alcohol here because you're using the fragrant tinctures you've made, which have 190-proof alcohol and some scent molecules dissolved in them. Because of the tincture's alcohol strength, you do not need a preservative or added alcohol to make the essential oils or absolutes soluble. You will, however, want to add some water to "lighten" the tincture and save some money because the tincture is pricey and time-consuming to make. I recommend adding only 3 percent of essential oils to the tincture spray to slightly deepen it and, of course, add to the scent complexity, making it a true perfume.

The following recipe makes about 8 ounces (237 ml).

MATERIALS AND EQUIPMENT

Beaker or graduated cylinder

Glass or stainless steel stirring rod or stainless steel skewer

Spray bottle, about 8–12 ounces (237–355 ml)

7 ml essential oils or absolutes (optional) (3 percent)

205 ml alcohol tincture (87 percent)

24 ml distilled water (10 percent)

Label and recordkeeping tools

PROCESS

1. Sterilize the beaker or cylinder, stirring rod or skewer, spray bottle, and spray top before adding any liquids (see "Safely Cleaning Equipment for Projects" on page 21, if needed).
2. Use the beaker or graduated cylinder to measure the liquids. In the bottle, combine the essential oils or absolutes, if using, and the tincture. Stir with the stirring rod. Wait for a moment for them to blend, then add the water.
3. Screw the spray top on, label the bottle, and you're ready to start using your natural, customized perfume!
4. Note that some tinctures and essential oils may stain. When using a linen spray, always test it on an inconspicuous part of the fabric before using it on the entire item. If you added essential oils or absolutes, you may need to shake the bottle each time before spraying because they will not dissolve completely. You can choose an opaque bottle if seeing the separate layers of the oil and waters is something you don't want.

Sweet Meadow Tincture Room and Linen Spray

1 ml lemongrass essential oil

3 ml bay laurel essential oil

3 ml vanilla absolute

205 ml alcohol tincture (use any tincture that has a light, soft fragrance, such as calendula, linden flower, lily, or sweet woodruff)

24 ml distilled water

Sensual Tincture Room and Linen Spray
(This blend is pricey, but so worth it!)

3 ml tuberose absolute

1 ml gardenia absolute

3 ml ambrette seed essential oil or absolute

205 ml alcohol tincture (a light woody or earthy tincture, such as sandalwood, patchouli, or sweetgrass, will blend well with the strong, sensual absolutes)

24 ml distilled water

SIMPLE BODY BUTTER WITH POMADE

Luxurious, silky, scented body butter is an indulgence that you will love—especially when it's 100 percent natural and you make it yourself. It's easy to make and requires few tools. The oils and pomades will nourish and protect your skin, and the fragrance you incorporate, either from an oil or pomade you've made or from the essential oils you add, will make it your personal signature scent. Because you don't add water, there is no need for a preservative.

This first recipe uses pomade that you've already made, or unscented shortening. On the next page, you'll find an alternate recipe. All of these recipes are somewhat interchangeable, and you can choose to use enfleurage pomade or regular shortening if you haven't made pomade yet. The choice of scent is up to you, and you may decide to make several different body butters by dividing the final whipped batch and adding different essential oils to each.

MATERIALS AND EQUIPMENT

1½ cups (360 ml) pomade or unscented shortening

Nonreactive bowl, such as glass, stainless steel, or enameled

1 cup (237 ml) coconut oil, infused fragrant oil, or oil of your choice

20–40 drops essential oils or absolutes

Hand or stand electric mixer

Spatula

Sterile jars for finished butter

Labels and record-keeping tools

PROCESS

1. Measure the pomade or shortening and place it in the bowl. Add the oil to the bowl. Finally, add the essential oils or absolutes.
2. Begin whipping the ingredients with the mixer on a low speed, gradually increasing to high speed.
3. During mixing, occasionally stop the mixer, and use a spatula to scrape the butter from the sides of the bowl. When the butter is soft and looks like whipped cream, stop the mixer and scrape it from the beaters.
4. Use the spatula to pack the butter into the jars. Place the lids on tightly, and label them.
5. Smoothing body butters onto your skin is a pleasant, sensual experience. I like to apply them after a shower, while my skin is still damp. They feel greasy for a few minutes but then soak in, leaving your skin very soft and gently perfumed. If you make a strong-scented body butter, you'll find it can be your perfume for that day, and you'll feel great, too, knowing your skin is soothed and nourished with the elegant butter.

Sleepy Time Sensual Body Butter

1½ cups (360 ml) fragrant floral pomade or unscented shortening

1 cup (237 ml) coconut oil, or an infused fragrant oil with a woodsy, warm scent, such as patchouli

20–40 drops essential oils or absolutes, such as vetiver, rose, lavender

Walk in the Garden Body Butter

1½ cups (360 ml) fragrant floral pomade or unscented shortening

1 cup (237 ml) coconut oil, or an infused fragrant oil with a sweet, floral scent, such as rose, ylang-ylang, orange blossom, honeysuckle, gardenia

20–40 drops essential oils or absolutes, such as rose, lavender, gardenia, orange blossom

TIP: When I store the body butters, I know in advance my house is too warm for them most of the time. My house is usually 78°F (26°C), and the butters become too soft, so I keep them in the refrigerator. They're still fine to use when stored at a higher temperature, but some of the height and fluff of the whip may deflate. Applying them chilled is a delightful experience, very cooling and soothing after a hot day. Be aware that moving them in and out of the refrigerator often and for extended times can pose a problem with condensation forming inside, and the water from the condensation can cause bacteria to grow. When I take a body butter from the fridge to remove some, I do it quickly so that the jar is back in the refrigerator in a minute or less.

ALTERNATE BODY BUTTER WITH VEGETABLE BUTTER

This body butter is made using a vegetable butter, such as mango or shea, along with either fixed oils or infused oils. Perhaps, if you haven't made a pomade yet but you have an infused fragrant oil, you can enjoy a body butter made with your infused oil and some essential oils.

MATERIALS AND EQUIPMENT

1 cup (237 ml) hard vegetable butter, such as mango, cocoa, or shea (may be mixed)

1 cup (237 ml) oil, such as infused oil you've made, or mixed with almond or coconut oil

Double boiler or glass bowl over saucepan that contains water

Spatula

Refrigerator

Spoon

20–40 drops essential oils or absolutes (optional)

Electric hand mixer, wire whisk, or egg beater

Jars

Label and recordkeeping tools

PROCESS

1. Add the vegetable butter and oil to the double boiler or nonreactive bowl, and place the container over moderately boiling water. Using a spatula, stir the mixture until the ingredients are melted and blended.
2. Remove the double boiler or bowl from the heat and allow it to cool to the touch. Place the container in the refrigerator and allow the mixture to harden. This is necessary to avoid crystallization as it cools, which can manifest as graininess in the butter.
3. After the butter hardens, remove it from the refrigerator and allow it to soften a bit, until you can move a spoon through it.
4. Add any essential oils or absolutes of your choice, if using.
5. Use a hand mixer, whisk, or egg beater to blend the butter again and incorporate the essential oils. Whip for about 15 minutes, or until it begins to fluff up in volume and get creamy.
6. Return to the refrigerator for 30 minutes to harden again.
7. Remove from the refrigerator and, working quickly, scoop the butter into jars. Seal and label them.

Chocolate Delight Body Butter Recipe

1 cup (237 ml) hard vegetable butter, such as cocoa butter

1 cup (237 ml) oil

20 drops chocolate essential oil or cocoa absolute

10 drops vanilla absolute

10 drops orange peel, peppermint, or spearmint essential oil, depending on your preferences

Wake Up! Body Butter Recipe

1 cup (237 ml) hard vegetable butter

1 cup (237 ml) oil, such as infused "green" type of oil you've made, including mint, rosemary, or Tagetes marigold, mixed with almond or coconut oil if you wish

20 drops mint essential oil

10 drops lemongrass essential oil

10 drops basil or lemon basil essential oil

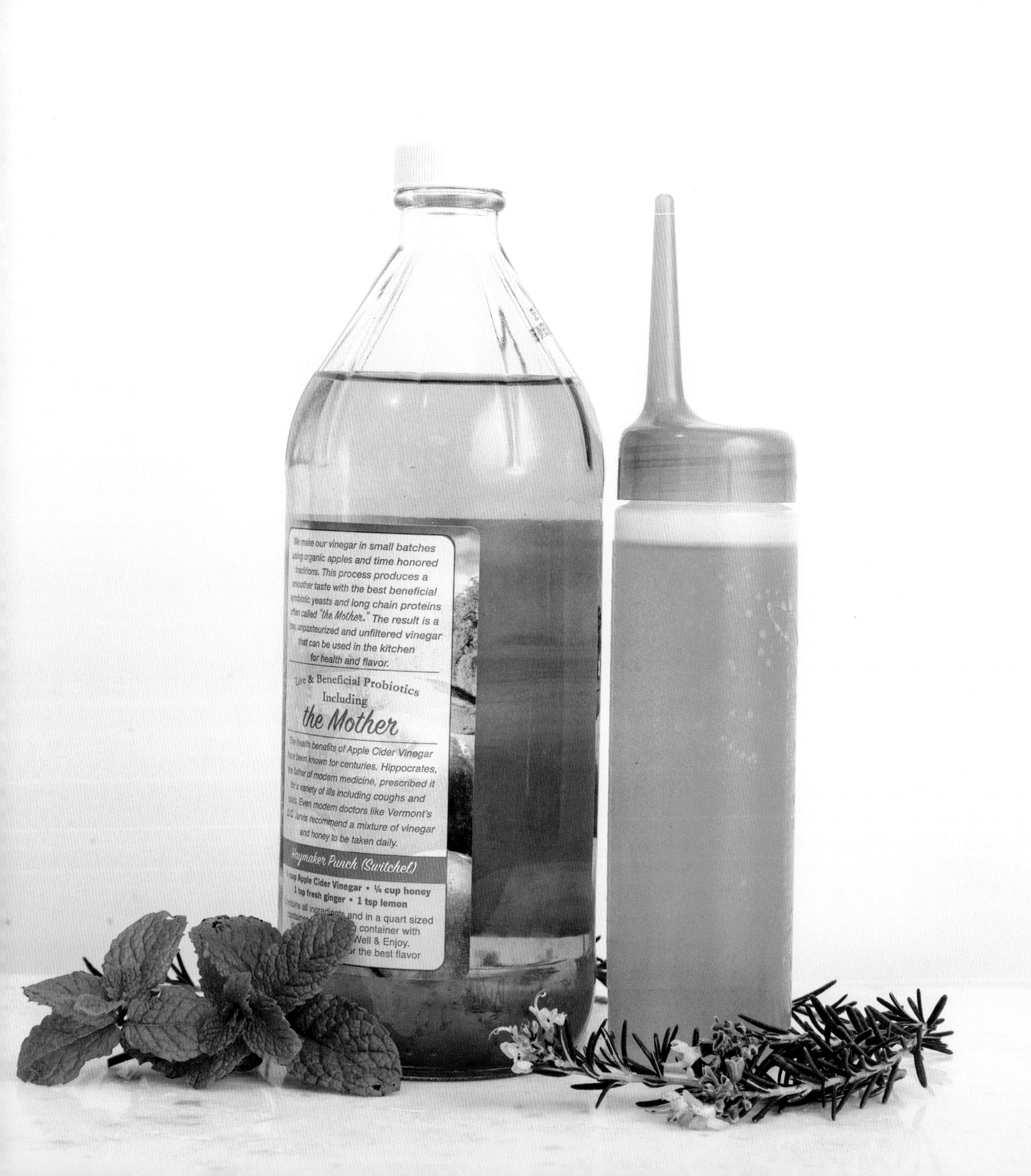
We make our vinegar in small batches using organic apples and time honored traditions. This process produces a smoother taste with the best beneficial symbiotic yeasts and long chain proteins often called "the Mother." The result is a raw, unpasteurized and unfiltered vinegar that can be used in the kitchen for health and flavor.
Live & Beneficial Probiotics Including
the Mother
The health benefits of Apple Cider Vinegar have been known for centuries. Hippocrates, the father of modern medicine, prescribed it for a variety of ills including coughs and colds. Even modern doctors like Vermont's D.C. Jarvis recommend a mixture of vinegar and honey to be taken daily.
Haymaker Punch (Switchel)
cup Apple Cider Vinegar • ¼ cup honey
1 tsp fresh ginger • 1 tsp lemon
and in a quart sized
container with
Well & Enjoy.
the best flavor

PERFUMED FACIAL, BODY, AND HAIR VINEGARS

Rose vinegar, made from rose petals and apple cider vinegar, is an excellent skin toner. Rose is the most common beauty vinegar, but others are discussed in "Introduction to Tincturing and Infusing" on page 26. Vinegars are good for your face, body, and hair. Their acidic nature helps restore the acid mantle of your skin, which can be adversely affected by alkaline water and soaps, the environment, and other factors. They are also antiseptic and antibacterial. Herbalists and others who make body products have known for centuries that a diluted vinegar rinse applied to the face, body, or hair can be beneficial. It will soften skin and make hair silky.

USING HERBAL VINEGARS

You need to dilute the finished vinegar with water before applying it to your skin or hair; never use vinegars undiluted. Follow the specific dilution instructions below for each application.

Always perform a patch test before using a new product on your face or body. Apply a small amount of the diluted mixture on the chin or behind the ear, and wait 24 hours to see whether there is a reaction in the form of an irritation or rash. If there is, do not use.

Basic recipe for your skin: Stir 2 tablespoons (30 ml) of the vinegar into 1 cup (237 ml) of pure water and follow the directions below for face and body.

For your face: Using cotton balls or a washcloth, gently dab the mixture onto your face. Allow to dry for 15 minutes, and rinse off with cool water.

For your body: Using the same ratio of 2 tablespoons (30 ml) per 1 cup (237 ml) of water, pour some of the mixture into your hands and splash it on your body. Allow to dry for 15 minutes, and rinse off with cool water.

For your hair: Dilute 2 ounces (60 ml) of vinegar with 6 to 8 ounces (177 to 237 ml) of water. After shampooing your hair, pour this dilution over it. Gently work it through with your fingers, squeezing it into the ends. Wait a few minutes, then rinse thoroughly. The vinegar acts as a clarifier, helping to remove residue of oils, dirt, shampoo, and any other product that may be lingering in your hair.

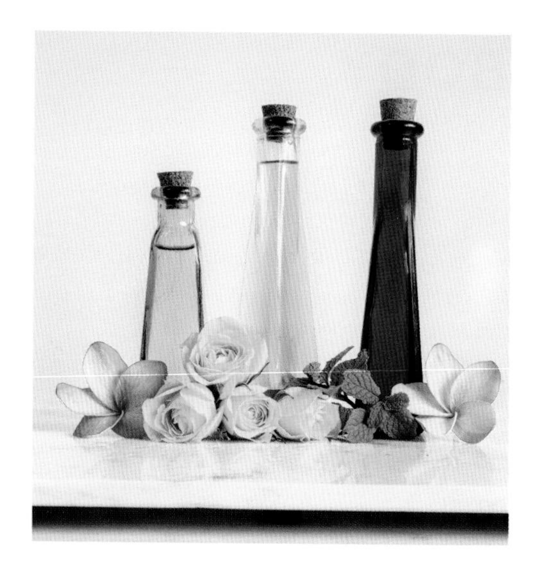

MASSAGE OILS

Blend light oils, such as almond and coconut, with a small percentage of essential oils or your infused oils. Blend several infused oils or essential oils in massage oil to create a custom scent. The botanicals from your infused oils provide healing properties to your massage oils, as well as scent.

PERFUMED HAIR OIL

Rich, emollient hair oils are even better when they contain natural fragrance. Use some of your infused oils for your hair, or make infusions specifically as hair oils. Perhaps you'd like to infuse the fragrance of roses or gardenias into a hair oil. Easy! Instead of using plain coconut oil for a hot oil treatment, you can blend some of your infusions into a custom-scented oil. Oils with a long shelf life, such as moringa, are good for this.

Using Hair Oil

Perfumed oils can be used to scent your hair, as well as condition it. If your hair is thick, you can apply a tiny bit as a hair perfume, applied near the roots, or underneath the back of your hair, near the nape of your neck. It's luxurious and sensual. You can apply your perfumed hair oils to the tips of your hair to scent it and to smooth and condition dry or flyaway ends. You can also apply them weekly to your entire head of hair for an intense hot-oil deep treatment.

PERFUMED POWDERS AND DEODORANT POWDERS

You can use scented enfleurage powder as body powder. Some powders can be used as a deodorant powder, especially when they contain myrrh and other base notes, such as frankincense. You may wish to mix a little finely powdered cinnamon, clove, sandalwood, and camphor wood with any enfleurage powder to mimic Asian *zukoh* powder, which is a traditional body/deodorant powder.

Put your powder in a shaker-top container, and apply it after shaking it into your hands. Or put it in a powder box with a soft, decadent powder puff.

PERFUMED BATH MILK

Bath milk is a wonderful way to perfume your bath while also adding moisturizing properties to the water. You need only a few ingredients to make this simple luxury. Use any of your oil infusions for this, either singly or blended. Add a single essential oil to the infused oil, or blend two or more to make a pleasing scent combination.

MATERIALS AND EQUIPMENT

2 cups (473 ml) whole milk or cream

1–2 tbsp (15–30 ml) infused oil

5–10 drops essential oil or absolute oil

Jar with a tight-fitting lid

PROCESS

1. Pour all of the ingredients into a covered jar and shake well before adding to a warm bath.
2. Climb in, relax, and enjoy your custom scent while the milk and oils moisturize your skin. Note: The tub may be slippery; use caution when getting out.
3. Use this bath milk immediately, or refrigerate for up to a week. If you'd like, you can use powdered whole milk instead of fresh milk, making sure to blend the oils well with the milk powder. This mixture will keep longer.

Relax and Restore Bath Milk

2 cups (473 ml) whole milk or cream

1–2 tbsp (15–30 ml) vetiver-, patchouli-, or sweetgrass-infused oil

5–10 drops spikenard and/or frankincense essential oil

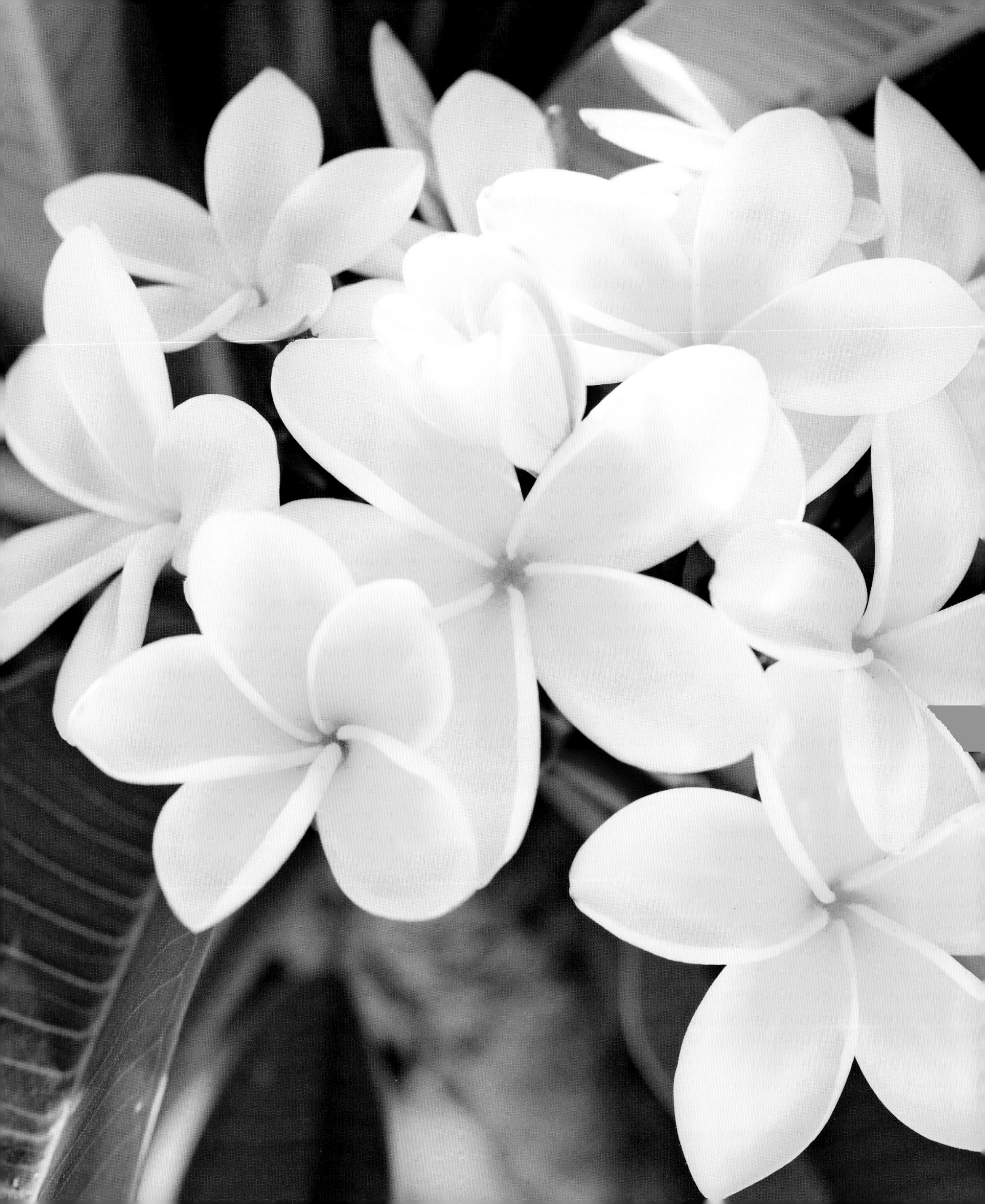

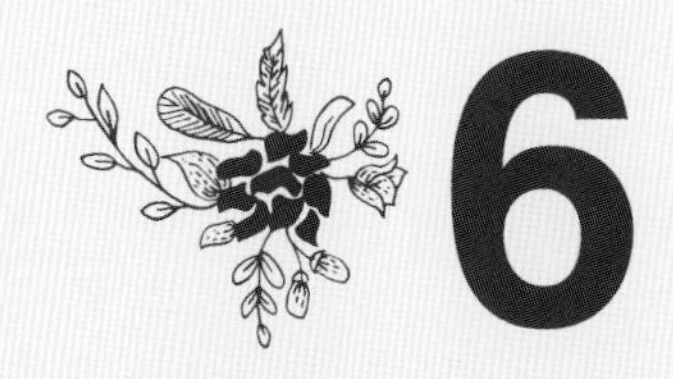

6

FRAGRANT PLANTS

This chapter contains briefs for 36 fragrant plants. Each brief gives both the common and botanical names for the plant, growing tips, perfumery uses, and a process chart so that you can decide which method to use to extract the scent. I selected a cross section of fragrant plants across many USDA growing zones. You may have plants in your garden that aren't listed, but use the information on a similar plant to begin your experimentation. Yields from the various extraction methods for each plant will vary. Most often with distillation, you'll obtain little essential oil but a lot of hydrosol. Tincturing may be the most rewarding extraction method. You can use the tinctures from most of the plants in this book in perfumes and in room and linen sprays. You can take the tincture a step further and evaporate or distill it to remove alcohol to obtain a beautiful oil absolute. Infusing yields pleasingly fragrant oils that have many uses, from simple face and body oils to solid perfumes and lip balms.

Left: Nothing says tropical fragrance like the beautiful frangipani, also known as plumeria, which blooms with many different scents, depending on the type. Some of mine smell like ripe peaches, coconut, tropical floral, citrus, and fruit mélange. If you don't live in the tropics or subtropics, you can grow them in pots and move them indoors in cold weather. *See page 145 for the full frangipani profile.*

CAUTION WITH FRAGRANT PLANTS

Not everything that smells pretty is safe to use for perfumery. Some plants contain substances that can be harmful if ingested, worn on skin, or inhaled; they can be allergens, irritants, or poisons. This book does not contain content on extracting the scent from harmful plants.

EXPLICIT WARNING: Never experiment with plants that are not listed in this book until you do research to ascertain that they are safe to extract and use for scent. You must research further to identify potential toxins, allergens, or irritants found in any of those plants. Additionally, if you know you're allergic to a specific plant, or plant family, do not experiment with extracting it.

PLANT SUBSTITUTION AND REGIONAL ADAPTATION

There are hundreds of plants worldwide that provide scent for extraction. This book covers only a good handful of them, but you can adapt my extraction guidelines when the plants are not found in this book (if you've researched the plant and found it to be safe).

Two different plants that grow in different USDA zones can have a similar scent. You can substitute extractions from plants in your area that smell similar to plants in this book that you can't grow where you live.

For example, orange jasmine (*Murraya paniculata*) and mock orange (*Philadelphus lewisii*) smell similar. You are not able to grow orange jasmine where you live, but mock orange does grow where you live. For extraction purposes, mock orange blossoms are similar in texture to another plant in this book, night-scented stock, which is extracted using tincturing Level 1, or infusing Level 2. This means the processing table for night-scented stock could be used for mock orange scent extraction.

Another example for substituting a plant not found in this book is Japanese snowbell (*Styrax japonicus*). You love its scent, and you know that it is safe to use extracts from the flowers, so you decide to extract its fragrance. Because Japanese snowbell flowers are similar in texture to lilac (*Syringa vulgaris*) flowers, the extraction process for lilac is suitable for these flowers.

AMBRETTE SEED, MUSK SEED

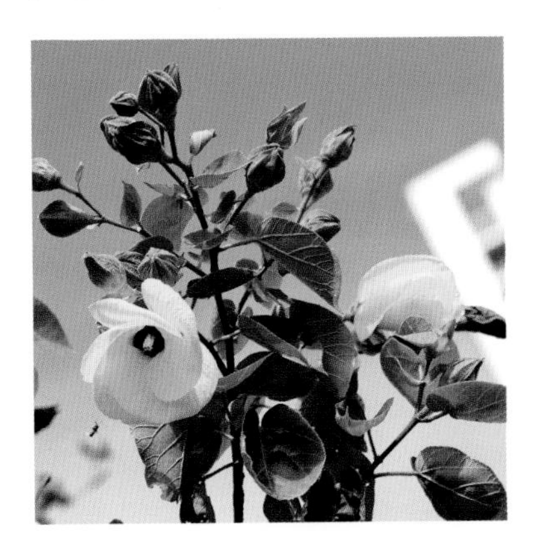

(Abelmoschus moschatus)

Perfumery: Base note

Related to hibiscus, this plant has large yellow flowers with a dark center, making it a beautiful ornamental. The seedpod may be unsightly, but the seeds are heavenly—a real treasure of beautiful fragrance.

There are two distinct scents you can get from ambrette seeds: The whole seeds smell sweet, fresh, musky, floral, uplifting, and buttery. The crushed seeds smell fatty; animalic, which most identify as musky; and deeply complex. The scent may develop a wine-like, or a port- or sherry-like, rich note.

GROWING GUIDELINES

This annual plant grows best in the summer season of zones 9b–11. It requires full sun, moderate watering, and well-drained soil. It's an easy plant to grow from seed. Sow directly in the ground in spring, and harvest the pods in fall.

Fifty plants will provide a substantial harvest, yielding approximately six seedpods per plant.

Note: If you aren't able to grow the plant, vendors sell seeds by the ounce (28 g) or the pound (454 g) for your perfumery purposes.

PREPARATION FOR PERFUMERY

Harvest when the pods are full and plump and the color is a rich green with a blush of red. Dry them at around 78°F (26°C), with low humidity and good ventilation. As soon as the pods are dry, break them open and remove the seeds.

PROCESS KEY

	TIME	NOTES
TINCTURE	Level 3. Up to 2 weeks to extract the seed scent. Shake the jar daily.	Historically, perfumers made a 25% tincture—that is, 25% seed to 75% solvent. Recharge two to three times, or more for a stronger-scented product.
INFUSION	Level 3. **Hot:** 48 hours or less, until saturation **Cold:** About 2 weeks, shaking frequently	See tincturing notes above. Hot infusing times vary greatly, from a few hours in a low-temperature double boiler to 24 to 48 hours for solar infusing, depending on the heat of the day and amount of direct sunlight.
DISTILLATION	Varies according to the distillation method and manufacturer's suggestion	Distill the uncrushed seeds. They may smell unpleasant for several months before developing a rich musk scent. Arctander advises to dilute the distillate 1:1 with high-proof alcohol after production to prevent an unpleasant fatty odor from developing.
ENFLEURAGE	N/A	Not a good enfleurage candidate because the seeds do not diffuse their scent well.

BALSAM FIR

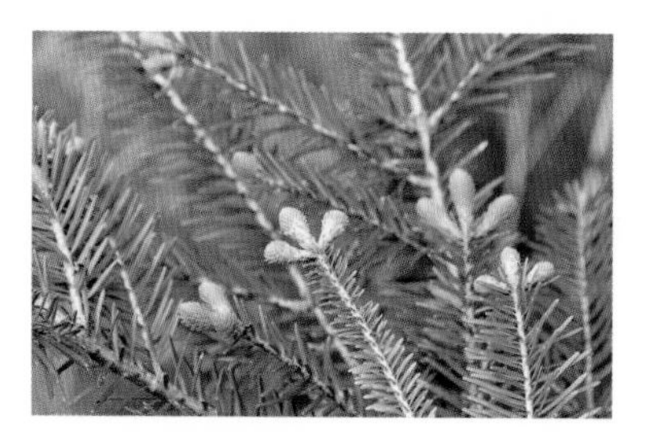

(Abies balsamea)

Perfumery: Middle note

The rich, round, resinous, balsamic, terpenic scent of balsam fir is among the most beloved of the conifers. For North American Christians, it is the smell of the Christmas tree. The trees' needles have a light, uplifting note. The resin is deep and rich, often described as "jammy" because it has some notes similar to those of cooked, ripe berries or plums.

The absolute is a thick, gummy substance with a most desirable scent for perfumery. The essential oil usually has a sharper, thinner scent than the absolute. Your extracts may fall somewhere between the two scents.

GROWING GUIDELINES

Although it grows mostly in the wild, if you live in zones 3–5, you may be able to grow it in your garden. This perennial evergreen tree can reach 50 feet (15 m) or more and grows in full sun.

Note: Your best source of the needles may be a recycled Christmas tree. One tree is enough for many projects.

PREPARATION FOR PERFUMERY

If you purchase a Christmas tree, get a balsam fir and don't discard the tree. Harvest the needles, buds (if there are any), and any resin on the bark. If you live in an area where they grow, you may be able to obtain fresh needles, buds, and resin. To save cleanup time, wear gloves to harvest. You can process the plant parts immediately, without drying them first.

PROCESS KEY

	TIME	NOTES
TINCTURE	Level 2. Two days, recharge as necessary.	Tincturing yields a strong-scented product. Leave the fir in the alcohol for 2 days; recharge with more material until scent is strong.
INFUSION	Level 2. **Hot:** 24 hours or less, until saturation **Cold:** A few hours to a few days	See tincturing notes above.
DISTILLATION	Varies according to the distillation method and manufacturer's suggestion	Balsam fir is easy to distill. Both the essential oil and hydrosol are evocative of the outdoors and fresh air.
ENFLEURAGE	N/A	Not suitable for enfleurage because they don't diffuse their scent well.

BAY LEAF, BAY LAUREL

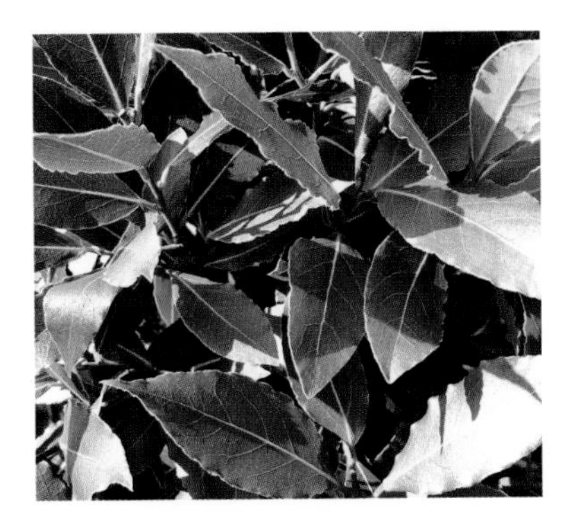

(Laurus nobilis)

Perfumery: Middle note

Bay leaf has an herbal, smooth, soft, moderately green, warm scent, reminiscent of thyme or oregano, but sweeter. It can also have notes that are fresh, camphorous, and slightly floral.

Bay leaf is used in perfumery, aromatherapy, and food flavoring. It plays a minor role in high-end perfumery, but a non-camphorous bay leaf oil, tincture, or infusion can provide a soft herbal note in clean, fresh, green perfumes.

GROWING GUIDELINES

An attractive perennial, it can be grown as a shrub or trained as a tree in zones 8–11. Protect the roots in colder climates. Purchase a plant, as seeds are very slow to germinate. Plant it in full sun to partial shade, and give moderate water in well-drained soil.

If you grow one vigorous bay leaf bush or tree at least 6 feet (2 m) tall, you should have a steady supply of leaves for extraction. It may take two years to reach that size, but you can harvest leaves in the meantime, as long as you don't strip the plant.

PREPARATION FOR PERFUMERY

You can use fresh or dried bay leaves. Harvest them when you see they have turned from soft, new leaves to fully mature, hard, stiff leaves.

PROCESS KEY

	TIME	NOTES
TINCTURE	Level 2. Two days. Recharge as necessary.	Tincturing is an efficient way to capture the scent of bay leaves quickly, and the scent is very true to that of the fresh leaf. Chop as directed for distillation. Do not tincture whole leaves.
INFUSION	Level 3. **Hot:** Up to 24 hours, or until saturation **Cold:** A few days	Bay leaf infusions can be used in making oil and solid perfumes. Chop as directed for distillation. Do not infuse whole leaves.
DISTILLATION	Varies according to the type of distillation and manufacturer's suggestion	Distillation yields little bay oil but a lot of hydrosol. Chop the leaves into small pieces. You can use a food processor for this, but do not overprocess the leaves into powder.
ENFLEURAGE	N/A	Bay leaves are not suited to enfleurage because they don't diffuse their scent well.

BUDDLEIA, BUTTERFLY BUSH

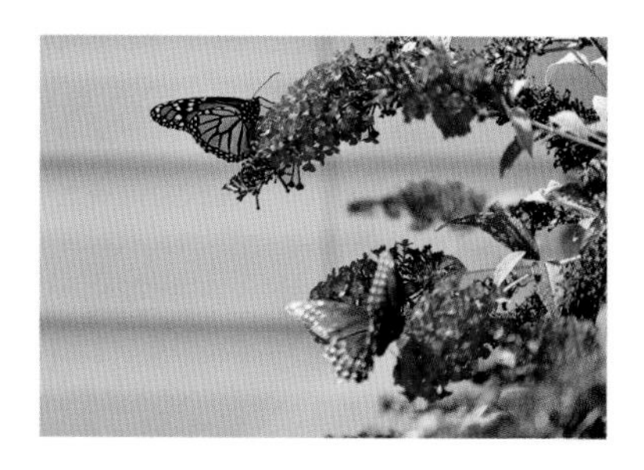

(*Buddleia davidii,* other spp.)

Perfumery: Middle note

Buddleia flowers have a soft, sweet, honey-like, powdery, floral scent. The large spikes of flowers resemble lilacs, and the plant is easy to grow.

GROWING GUIDELINES

This carefree perennial does best in zones 5–10 and can reach 4 to 20 feet (1 to 6 m), depending on the species. In the hot, humid South, it's best to plant in the fall. It likes full sun and moderate water with well-drained soils. It may be grown in containers and is easy to grow from cuttings. Flowers range in color from white to almost black, including peach, yellow, red, bicolor, blue, purple, lavender, and pink. It attracts butterflies, hummingbirds, and bees.

Buddleias are generous bloomers, and a midsize bush of 6 to 8 feet (2 to 2.5 m) will provide many flower spikes for most projects.

PREPARATION FOR PERFUMERY

Harvest the fully mature and opened flower heads and process immediately. You may wilt them slightly if you determine they are very moist.

PROCESS KEY

	TIME	NOTES
TINCTURE	Level 1. Up to 24 hours, or until saturation	Tinctures very well; requires several recharges to reach desired scent strength.
INFUSION	Level 2. **Hot:** 24 hours or less, or until saturation **Cold:** A few hours to a few days	Cold or hot infusion. Good for making oil or solid perfumes.
DISTILLATION	Varies according to distillation method and manufacturer's suggestion	Distillation yields a sweetly perfumed hydrosol but very little oil.
ENFLEURAGE	Until petals turn translucent, start to brown, or no longer give off scent	Excellent for large-container enfleurage.

CALENDULA, MARIGOLD, POT MARIGOLD

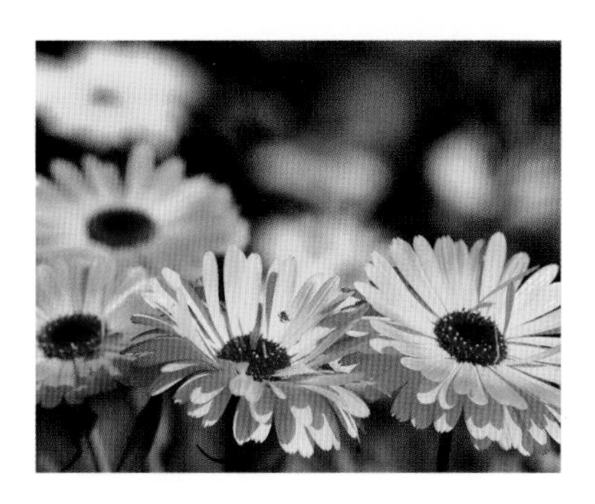

(Calendula officinalis)

Perfumery: Middle note

The rich, strong-scented floral note of the cheerful orange or yellow calendula flowers is clean and light. There are warm, honey-like tones and a bit of crisp greenness. Refreshing.

All parts of the plant are sticky with fragrant resin. Don't confuse it with another plant called marigold, *Tagetes* spp. (See the plant brief for marigold on page 164.)

GROWING GUIDELINES

Sow the seeds of this annual in a sunny area early in the spring, but if you are in a hot, humid climate, then grow it as a winter crop. The plants can grow as large as 3 feet (90 cm) tall and 2 feet (60 cm) wide, depending on the species. Cut the blooms when they are fully open, and new flowers will replace them. It needs moderate water and well-drained soil.

Grow at least 100 plants for a plentiful harvest. The flower heads are generously yielding of their scent and color, and a few go a long way.

PREPARATION FOR PERFUMERY

Pick the fully opened flowers after the morning dew evaporates, and let the flowers wilt slightly before processing. Do not let them dry because it diminishes the scent.

PROCESS KEY

	TIME	NOTES
TINCTURE	Level 1. 24 hours, or until saturation	Tincturing yields a very herbal product with floral tones. Recharge for scent intensity, as desired.
INFUSION	Level 2. **Hot:** A few hours, or until saturation **Cold:** A few hours to a few days	Exceptional skin oil
DISTILLATION	Varies according to the distillation method and manufacturer's suggestion	You will obtain a little oil and a sweet hydrosol that is wonderful for the skin.
ENFLEURAGE	Until petals turn translucent, start to brown, or no longer give off scent.	Calendulas can be used in both large-container and traditional enfleurage. They don't have a lot of scent to diffuse but can make a soft, subtle pomade.

CARNATION, DIANTHUS, CLOVE PINKS

(Dianthus caryophyllus)

Perfumery: Top to middle note

Carnation flowers have a fresh, floral, spicy note that many people describe as cheerful and clean. They share scent chemicals in common with cloves and are often called clove pinks. Several species of *Dianthus* are fragrant and well known, including sweet William (*D. barbatus*) and pinks (*D. plumarius*).

GROWING GUIDELINES

Carnations can grow up to 3 feet (1 m) tall and come in many colors, including white, pink, red, and yellow. Confirm when buying seeds or plants online that it is a strong-scented variety. They grow easily in zones 5–9, in full sun with moderate water and good drainage. Cut the flowers to encourage new flowers to bloom.

PREPARATION FOR PERFUMERY

Start with two dozen plants or so. Carnations can vary so greatly in size that it's difficult to predict what you will need for a project. If you can't grow enough to supply your needs, you can buy them at wholesale markets.

Use garden scissors to snip the blossoms carefully from the stems. Remove the green calyx at the base of each flower. Process flowers immediately, or allow them to wilt slightly for an hour or two in a shady, cool spot.

PROCESS KEY

	TIME	NOTES
TINCTURE	Level 1. 24 hours, or until saturation	May need many recharges to obtain a strong scent.
INFUSION	Level 2. **Hot:** 24 hours or less, or until saturation **Cold:** A few hours to a few days	May need many recharges to obtain a strong scent. Wilt slightly before extracting. Check carefully for water and mold; discard if found. Recharging hot infusions may cause degradation of scent and oil.
DISTILLATION	Varies according to distillation method and manufacturer's suggestion	Distillation yields a spicy, floral hydrosol but very little oil. The hydrosol makes a clove-type-scented room or linen spray. Makes a refreshing body spray.
ENFLEURAGE	Until petals turn translucent, start to brown, or no longer give off scent	Carnations are good candidates for large-container enfleurage.

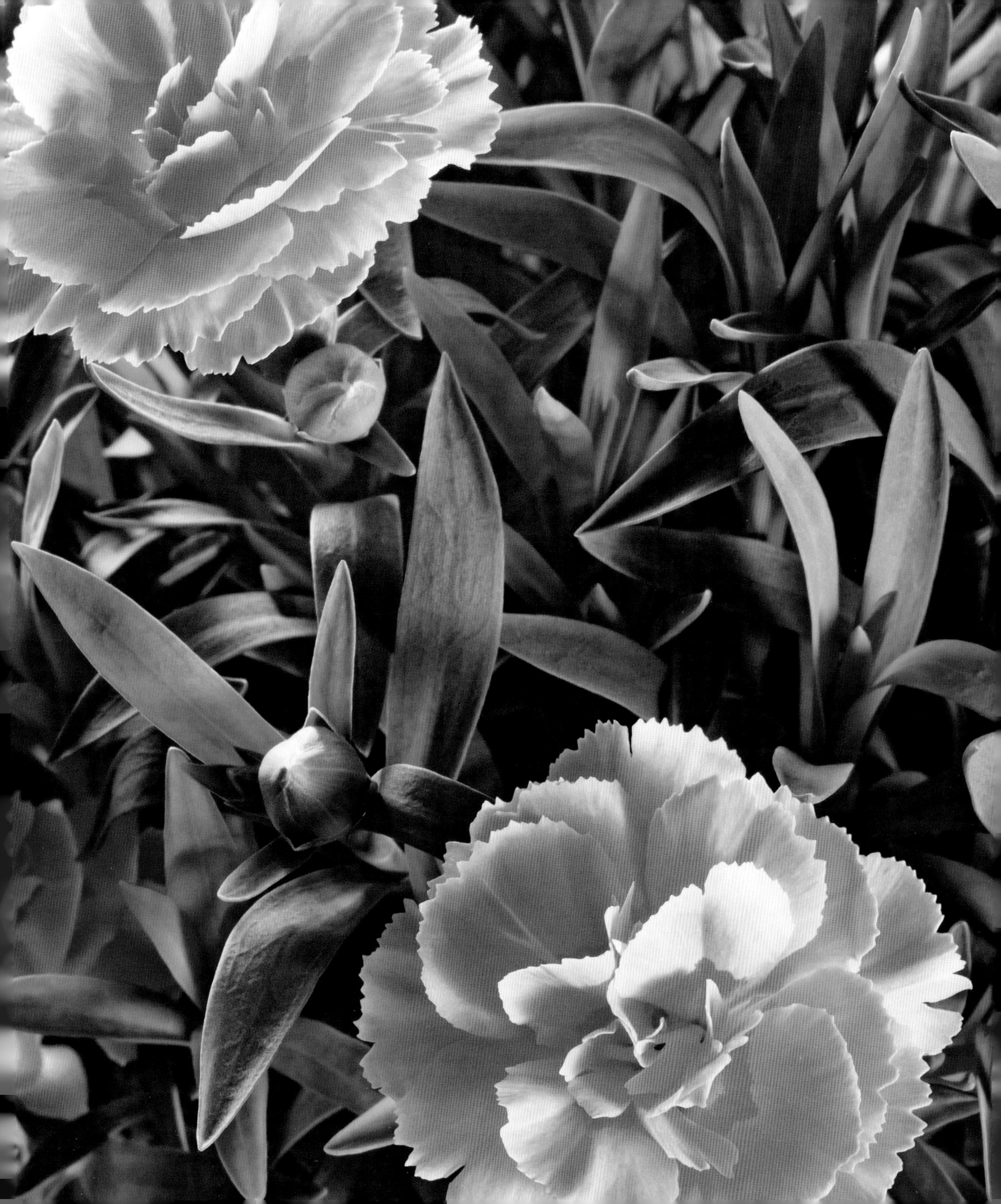

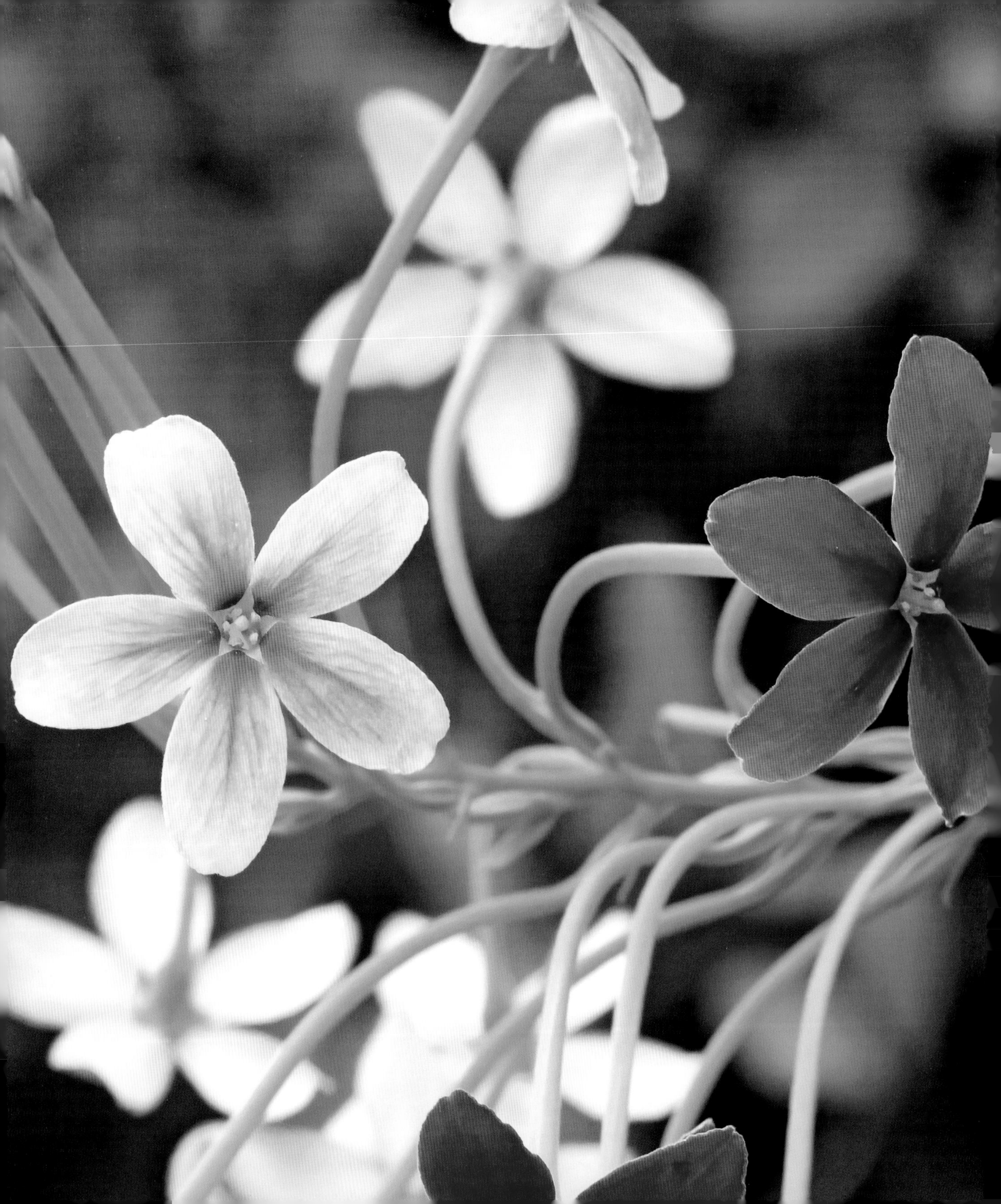

CHINESE HONEYSUCKLE, RANGOON CREEPER

(Quisqualis indica)

Perfumery: Middle note

This is a sweet floral, somewhat like jasmine flower with a toasted coconut note. It has an inviting tropical flower scent. It has been called hypnotic because it can overwhelm you with its scent.

Quisqualis is an aggressive vine. There are single- and double-flowered varieties. Whether single or double, the showy flower clusters are a conversation piece in the garden. The flowers open white, turn pink, then red and can be viewed concurrently on one spray, which is very attractive.

GROWING GUIDELINES

If you live north of zones 10 and 11, you may still get a nice crop of flowers if you obtain a plant through mail order in early spring and give it a fence or trellis to climb on. You should get many successive blooms before frost. In zones 10–11, it is a perennial, growing up to 40 feet (12 m) in one season. It likes full sun to partial shade, moderate water, and well-drained soil.

A small plant will grow into a large vine in one season. One plant will yield enough flowers for several extract processes.

PREPARATION FOR PERFUMERY

Harvest a flower cluster with a mix of white, pink, and red flowers for optimum scent. Observe what time of day the flowers are the most fragrant; they may be extremely fragrant in the evening.

PROCESS KEY

	TIME	NOTES
TINCTURE	Level 1. 24 hours, or until saturation	With many recharges, tincturing yields a strong-scented product.
INFUSION	Level 2. Varies	Infusing takes the same dedication and time as tincturing. Cold infusing is the best option because you'll need a lot of recharges, and repeatedly heating up the oil will degrade the infusion. Many other flowers can withstand hot infusions, but Chinese honeysuckle flowers are so tiny, the repetitions necessary challenge the efficacy of it.
DISTILLATION	Varies according to the distillation method and manufacturer's suggestion	Yields a sweetly floral hydrosol but very little oil.
ENFLEURAGE	Until petals turn translucent, start to brown, or no longer give off scent	A good candidate for large-container enfleurage. The flowers are very delicate and may wilt in the container, so you may have to remove them after 6 hours and recharge the fat.

CITRUS—ORANGE, LEMON, LIME, GRAPEFRUIT, EXOTICS

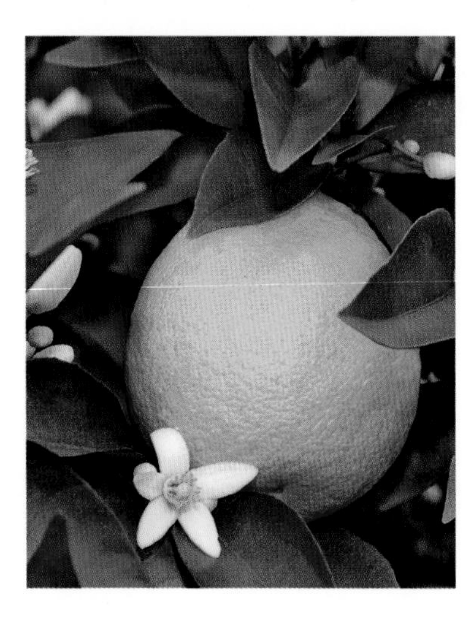

(Citrus sinensis, C. limon, C. paradisi)

Perfumery: Citrus rind essential oils are top notes. The flowers, leaves, and stems are top to middle notes.

There are many types of citrus fruits, and they all have a similarity—they're zesty, refreshing, and bright, with a fruity scent and flavor—yet they are very different from each other. In perfumery, in addition to the rind oils of many citruses used, the leaves (called *petitgrain*) and flowers of several species are also extracted.

Caution: Several citruses, especially limes, grapefruits, and bergamot oranges, are phototoxic, reacting upon skin when it's exposed to sunlight, and causing berlock dermatitis. I urge perfume gardeners to research any citrus oil that you're using to determine the safest percentage for your specific product.

GROWING GUIDELINES

These perennial tropical and subtropical plants thrive outdoors in zones 8–11, depending on the species. They also can be grown in containers and moved indoors in colder climates. They need full sun, moderate water, and well-drained soil and are easy to grow.

Citrus leaves may be the most rewarding part of the tree to process because of their abundance. One small outdoor or container tree can provide enough material for extraction. Tincturing and infusing the flowers and leaves, and the peeled rinds, if you wish to try that, can give immediate gratification and a great product. You can keep the tincture and infusions in a cool, dark place and add successions of recharges as necessary to reach the scent intensity you desire.

PREPARATION FOR PERFUMERY

Citrus flowers are best harvested just after they open. Keep in mind that if you remove most, or all, of the flowers, you won't get fruits. The leaves and/or branch tips can be clipped from the tree at any time, and if there are small, immature fruits on the branches, all the better, because this will give you the true petitgrain.

PROCESS KEY		
	TIME	**NOTES**
TINCTURE	**Flowers:** Level 1. Up to 24 hours, or until saturation **Leaves:** Level 2. 1 day **Rind:** Levels 2–3. 1 day, up to several days	Tinctures of citrus parts are rewarding. Leaves and rinds should be slightly dried, then chopped before processing.
INFUSION	**Flowers:** Level 2. Until it becomes translucent—could be only 1 minute **Leaves:** Level 2. 1 day **Rind:** Levels 2–3. 1 day, up to several days	Experiment with all three fragrant parts of the citrus tree and create oil or solid perfumes.
DISTILLATION	Varies according to the distillation method, part of plant used, and manufacturer's suggestion	Flowers yield a beautiful hydrosol and a little oil. Leaves are easy to distill. Wilt them for a few hours and chop into small pieces first. Fruits yield a bright, "foodie" hydrosol and a little oil.
ENFLEURAGE	Until petals turn translucent, start to brown, or no longer give off scent	Only the citrus flowers are suitable for enfleurage because they diffuse their scent into the fat. Use the large-container enfleurage method, placing flowers in a mesh bag or on a wire cooling rack or a screen, suspended above the fat. Otherwise, the flowers can stick to the fat and fall apart when you try to remove them.

CORIANDER SEED

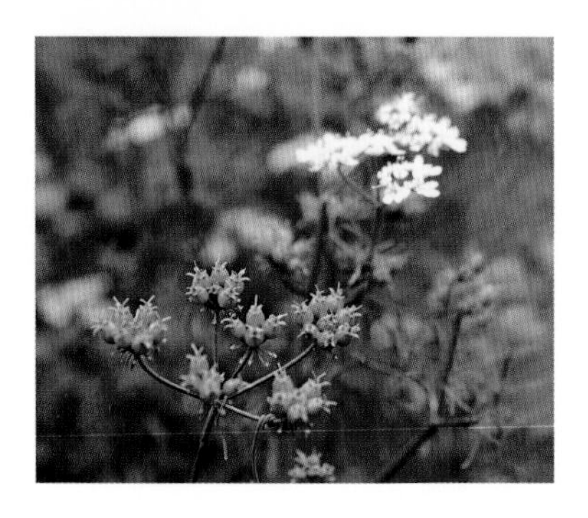

(Coriandrum sativum)

Perfumery: Top note

This small seed has a complex odor profile: It smells a bit like sage and is spicy, sweet, herbaceous, fruity, woody, lemon-citrusy, and pungent. Coriander seed is a valued top note in natural perfumery. It is uplifting and enticing, blending well with many other aromatics. The leaves of the plant are known as cilantro, and they have a completely different scent, which some people, if they carry a specific gene, describe as "soapy" and unpleasant.

GROWING GUIDELINES

This annual herb can be grown in all zones and, aside from the hot South, is best grown starting in the spring. It must be sown after danger of frost is past. It grows to about 18 inches (46 cm) tall and likes full sun to partial shade and consistent watering. Do not allow it to dry out.

Note: If you aren't able to grow the plant, vendors sell seeds by the ounce (28 g) or the pound (454 g) for perfumery purposes.

PREPARATION FOR PERFUMERY

Harvest the seeds when they turn yellow or brown and have distinct longitudinal ridges. Cut the seed heads off the stalk, using a small basket under them to catch ones that may drop. They can be processed immediately or dried for later processing. If your harvest is small, you can purchase coriander seeds and use them instead to supplement your harvest.

PROCESS KEY

	TIME	NOTES
TINCTURE	Level 2. Several hours to 2 days	Tincturing yields a sweet-scented top-note product. Recharge the tincture until you achieve the scent intensity you want.
INFUSE	Level 3. **Hot:** A few hours **Cold:** A few hours to a few days	Coriander oil is strong and spicy. Can be used for oil and solid perfumes.
DISTILLATION	Varies according to the distillation method and manufacturer's suggestion	Presoaking the seeds in water increases the essential oil yield. Distillation yields approximately one-half of 1% oil by weight.
ENFLEURAGE	N/A	The coriander seed does not diffuse enough fragrance to be a good candidate for enfleurage.

FRANGIPANI, PLUMERIA

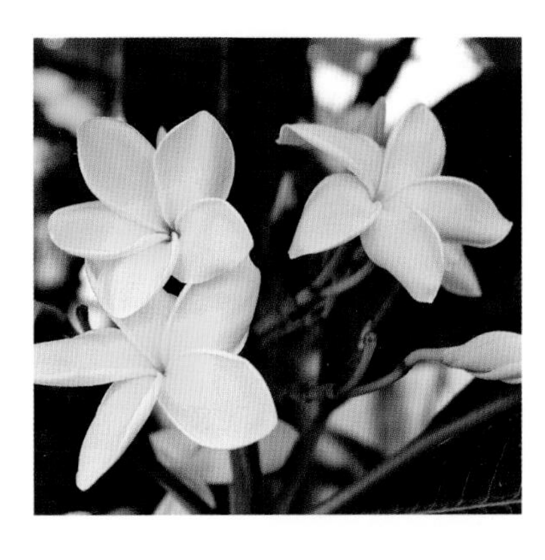

(Plumeria alba, P. rubra)

Perfumery: Middle note

The most common frangipani scent is warm, jasmine-like, floral, and buttery, with perhaps a touch of fruit. Various frangipanis can smell like citrus, spice, peaches, apricots, and bubblegum. Flowers are most fragrant at night. The frangipani flowers are often made into Hawaiian leis.

Frangipanis are related to oleanders and are native to Central and South America. They are also called plumeria, their genus name, but perfumers use the term frangipani. The white sap may be an irritant if you get it into your eyes or mouth, but it washes off easily.

GROWING GUIDELINES

Grow outdoors in zones 10–11, and in colder climates, grow in pots to move indoors. This perennial is slow growing, and the yield can vary from scant to plentiful, depending on care and feeding and variety. It can grow to 20 feet (6 m) and is deciduous. It likes full sun and minimal water and can withstand drought conditions.

PREPARATION FOR PERFUMERY

You can harvest enough flowers to process from one midsize plant (6 feet [2 m]). Enfleurage is probably the optimum way to extract their scent if you have limited flowers because it requires fewer recharges to obtain a strong-scented product than the other methods.

Pick the flowers in the early evening, when their fragrance has developed. Break off the flower at the stem. Be careful not to bruise or crush the flowers. Allow them to wilt slightly for no more than an hour.

PROCESS KEY

	TIME	NOTES
TINCTURE	Level 1. Up to 24 hours, or until saturation	Requires numerous recharges to obtain a strong-scented tincture.
INFUSION	Level 2. **Hot:** 1 hour or less **Cold:** A few hours to a few days	Hot infusion is best because of the watery nature of the flower. Cold infusions can rot more easily. Wilt the flowers for an hour or two to evaporate some of the water from them and to dry the latex on the cuts.
DISTILLATION	Varies according to the distillation method and manufacturer's suggestion	Can yield a beautifully sweet hydrosol. Wilt flowers for an hour or two before distilling.
ENFLEURAGE	Until petals turn translucent, start to brown, or no longer give off scent	Suitable for traditional enfleurage or large-container enfleurage.

GARDENIA—AMERICAN, TAHITIAN, VIETNAMESE

(*Gardenia jasminoides* [American], *G. tahitensis* [Tahitian, Tiare], *G. vietnamensis* [genus syn. Kailarsenia])

Perfumery: Middle note

Related to coffee (which also has fragrant flowers), *Gardenia jasminoides* is the flower best known to Americans, but gardenias from Tahiti and Vietnam are also lovely for perfume. *G. jasminoides* has a warm, narcotic floral scent, with butter and milk notes, similar to jasmine but much rounder and richer. *G. tahitensis* is fruitier than any other gardenias. Soft and sweetly floral, this is the gardenia of the famous Monoi scent. I grow the double-flowered variety. *G. vietnamensis* is a bold, strong, spicy floral, but the scent doesn't diffuse far. It blooms year-round with striking pinwheel-looking flowers. You may detect some notes in common with ylang-ylang and coconut, depending on the variety and time of day.

GROWING GUIDELINES

This perennial shrub with shiny leaves and big flowers grows in zones 8–11 but can be grown in pots and moved indoors in northern zones. It likes full sun and consistent water, as drying out can cause the buds to drop.

Gardenias are so full of scent that even one blossom is a good candidate for a cup or large-container enfleurage. If you have a large plant, or a number of plants, I recommend large-container enfleurage. Many wholesale flower companies will sell slightly imperfect *G. jasminoides* gardenia "seconds" at a good discount. There is nothing wrong with them other than their aesthetic quality; they may be lopsided or missing a few petals.

PREPARATION FOR PERFUMERY

Wait until the buds are fully open, and they will continue to produce scent for several days. Harvest when the dew or rain is dried from the flowers, and take care not to bruise the fleshy petals. Let them wilt for a few hours before processing.

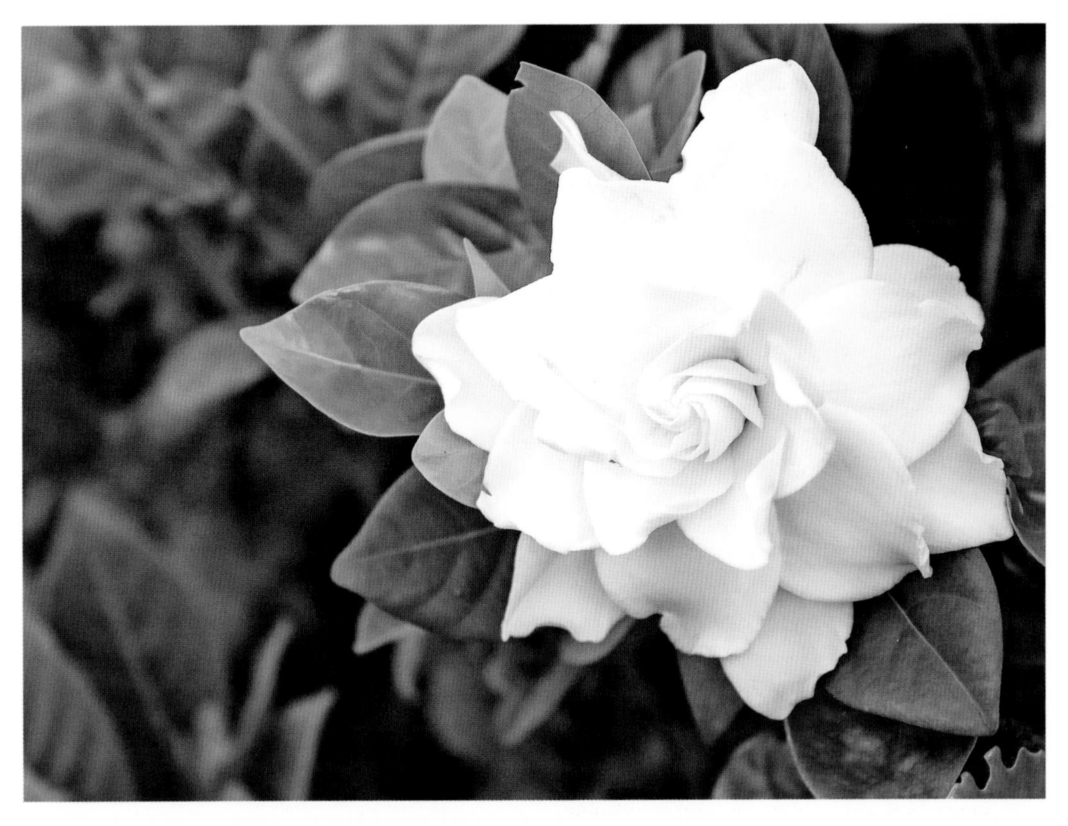

PROCESS KEY		
	TIME	**NOTES**
TINCTURE	Level 1. Up to 24 hours, or until saturation	Tincturing gardenia is very rewarding. Recharge the tincture until you obtain the desired scent intensity.
INFUSION	Level 2. **Hot:** 1 hour or less	Hot infusion is recommended because of the watery nature of the flower. If it's cold infused, it may rot.
DISTILLATION	Varies according to the distillation method and manufacturer's suggestion	Distillation yields very little oil but a lot of hydrosol.
ENFLEURAGE	Until petals turn translucent, start to brown, or no longer give off scent	A very rewarding enfleurage flower, whether you have one or many. A pomade-lined cup with a lid can extract the scent from one.

HONEYSUCKLE

(*Lonicera japonica,* other spp.)

Perfumery: Middle note

The rambling honeysuckle vine is a sweet, floral summertime delight. It has a touch of honey, orange flower, fatty, creamy notes, and a bit of the exotic zing of tuberose. The showy flowers are very fragrant and come in a variety of colors. Very decorative.

GROWING GUIDELINES

Grows in zones 8–11. Evergreen vine, sometimes shrub. Shrubs grow to 6 feet (3 m) to 15 feet (4.5 m), vines up to 20 feet (6 m). Invasive, but can be controlled by pruning. Blooms spring through summer.

One large vine or shrub will provide you with an abundance of flowers. You may also harvest wild honeysuckle, or some from an agreeable neighbor, to augment your extraction. You may plant two or more honeysuckles and have an overabundance, but that's nothing to complain about because it's so delightful and easy to process.

PREPARATION FOR PERFUMERY

Morning dew may help the scent permeate the air, and you may wish to harvest then. If you do, be sure to let the dew dry off before processing. When the temperature is above 85°F (29°C), the scent may diminish. Scent is typically stronger at night, so you may harvest at dusk or nightfall if that suits you. As they are slightly wilting before processing, the scent will continue to get stronger, as if they were still on the vine or shrub.

PROCESS KEY

	TIME	NOTES
TINCTURE	Level 1. Up to 24 hours, or until saturation	Wilt the flowers for an hour or two, and recharge when they noticeably lose color or turn translucent.
INFUSION	Level 2. **Hot:** 1 hour or less **Cold:** A few hours to a few days	Wilt the flowers for an hour or two to evaporate some of the water before infusing them.
DISTILLATION	Varies according to the distillation method and manufacturer's suggestion	Distillation yields very little oil, but a lot of hydrosol. May be a good candidate for co-distillation, with lemon or rose or other fragrant harvests that will stand up to the honeysuckle's strong scent.
ENFLEURAGE	Until petals turn translucent, start to brown, or no longer give off scent	A very rewarding enfleurage flower. It's a good candidate for either traditional or large-container enfleurage, as well as maceration.

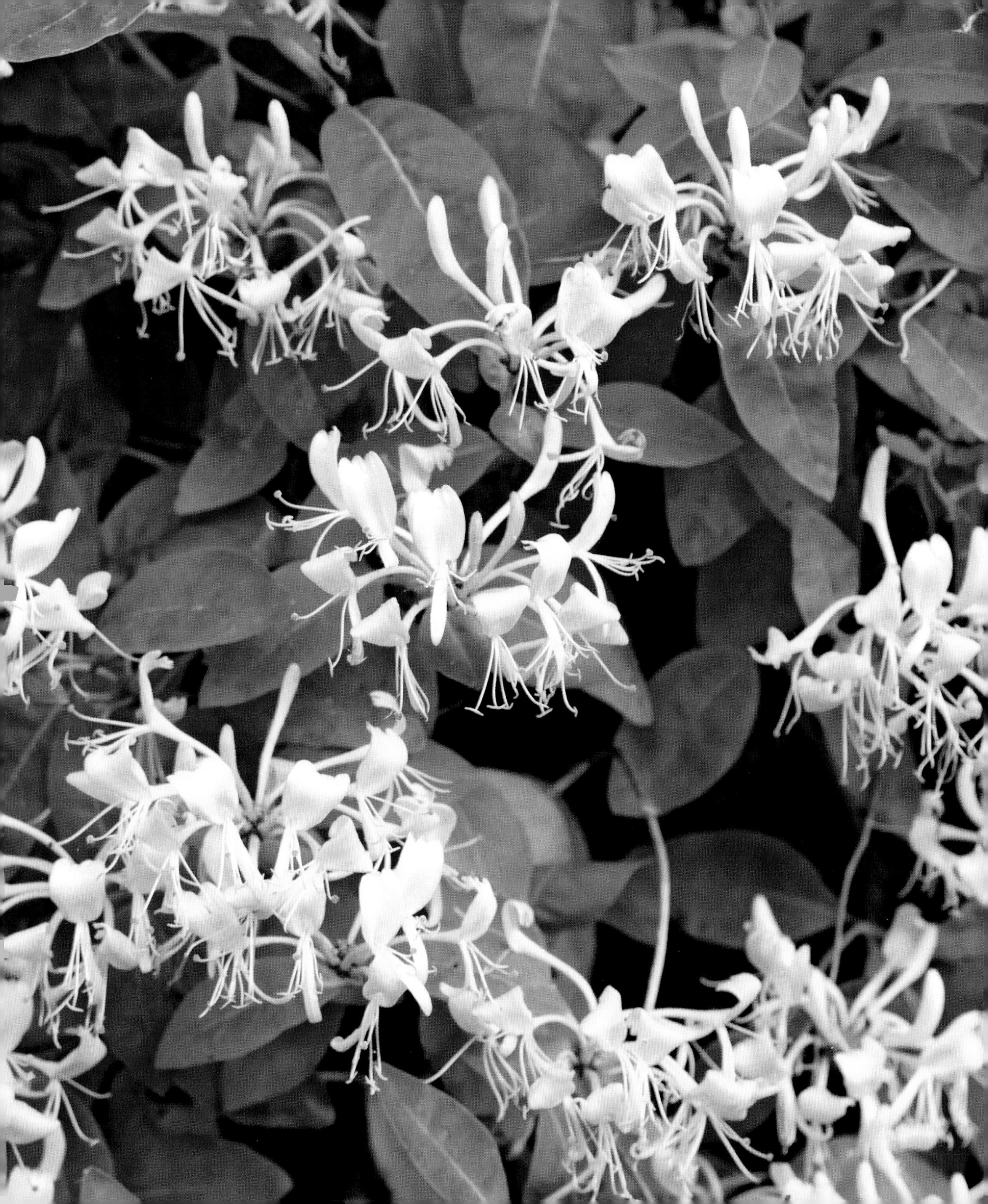

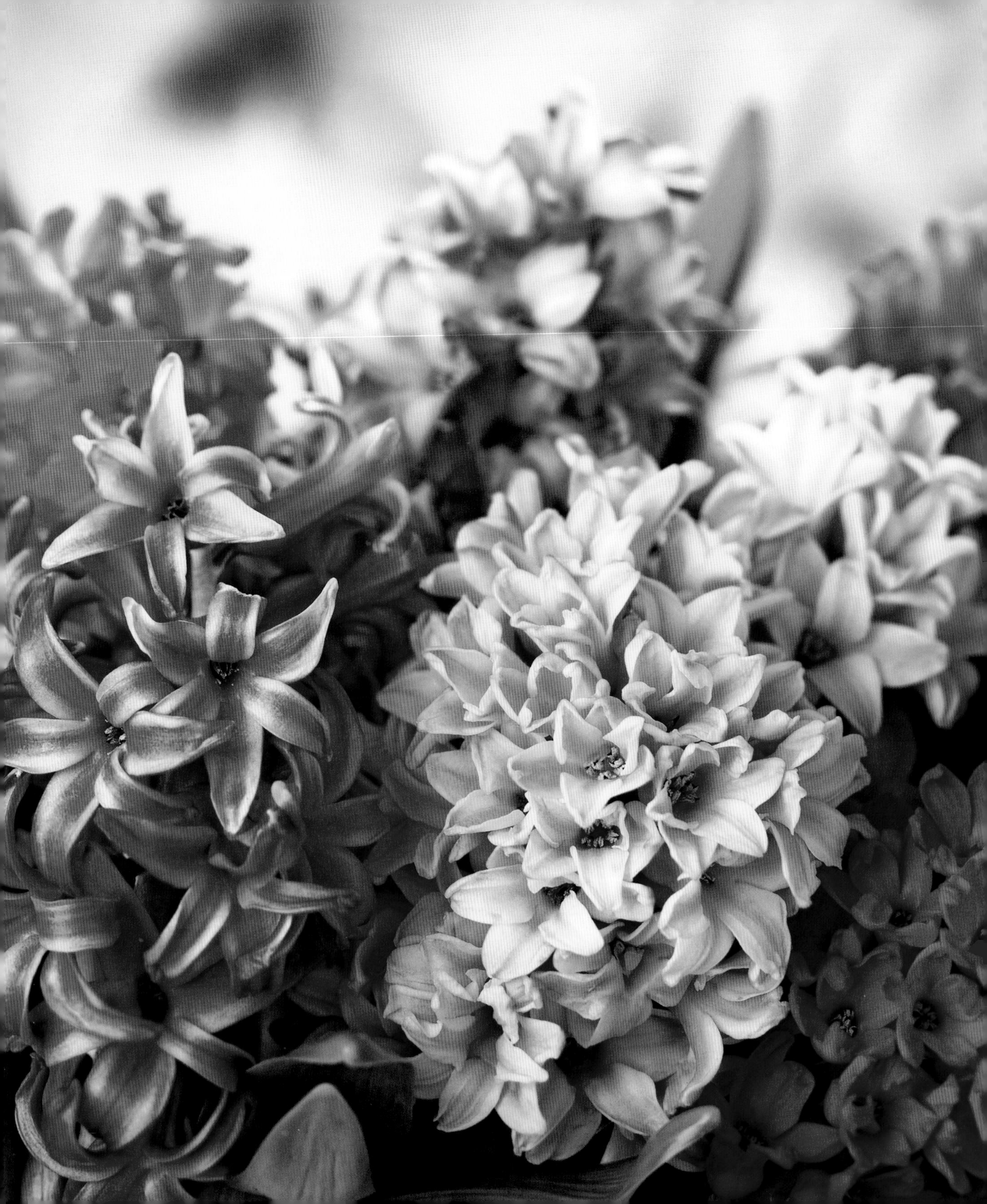

HYACINTH

(*Hyacinthus orientalis,* other spp.)

Perfumery: Middle note

The pretty purple, pink, or white hyacinth flowers have a sharp, intoxicating, almost overpowering sweet, cool green floral scent with spicy cinnamon tones, and an airy diffusive character. Some say it "tickles" your nose because of its spicy scent; others may find it a bit soapy. The hyacinth is a spring flowering bulb in the Northern Hemisphere that is native to Turkey and the eastern Mediterranean shores. Once established in a garden, hyacinth bulbs spread and multiply, providing visual and fragrant delight when they bloom.

GROWING GUIDELINES

These perennial bulbs may be purchased already "forced"—that is, having received cold storage preparation for planting in warmer climates. They thrive in zones 6–8 and require full sun, moderate water, and well-drained soil. The flowering top growth rarely exceeds 12 inches (30 cm) in height and can be massed in the planting bed. They will reproduce by side bulbs. Two dozen flowers will provide several recharges for extraction. If you live in the hyacinth-growing region, you may have a generous garden harvest and can proceed accordingly. If you live in very cold or hot climates, you can purchase the bulbs in bloom from specialty stores or wholesalers.

PREPARATION FOR PERFUMERY

Cut the flower spike at the base after all of the florets have completely opened. Lay the flower spikes on their side in a cool, dark place and allow them to wilt for a few hours before processing. You may also wish to remove the individual florets from the central stem.

PROCESS KEY

	TIME	NOTES
TINCTURE	Level 1. 24 hours, or until saturation	Tincture the individual florets rather than the whole flower head.
INFUSION	Level 2. **Hot:** 1 hour or less. **Cold:** A few hours to a few days	Wilt the flowers for an hour or two to evaporate some of the water from them before infusing. Snip the florets from the stem before infusing; don't infuse the stem. In cold infusion, remove the flowers before they begin to get moldy. If you find the slightest sign of mold, discard the entire infusion and start over.
DISTILLATION	Varies according to the distillation method and manufacturer's suggestion	Distillation yields very little oil but a lot of hydrosol
ENFLEURAGE	Until petals turn translucent, start to brown, or no longer give off scent	A very rewarding enfleurage flower and a good candidate for either traditional or large-container enfleurage. Cutting the individual florets off the spike for traditional enfleurage may result in mold, as a result of the water released, so let them wilt for an hour or more to discourage that. Large-container enfleurage, in which the florets can remain attached to the stem, helps prevent mold. It's a good enfleurage maceration flower as well. Remove individual florets from the stem, and discard the stem.

JASMINE

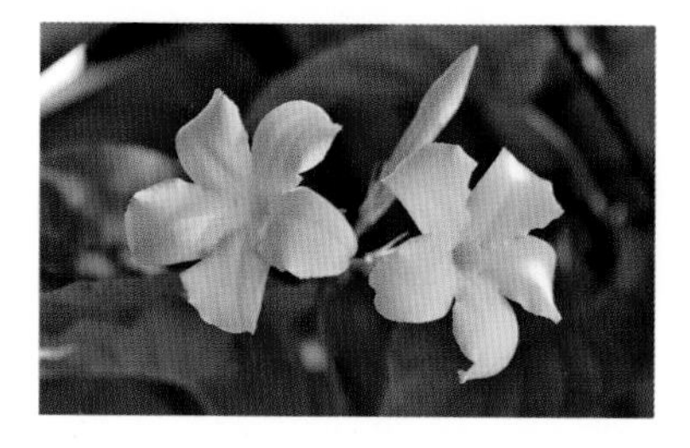

(Jasminum grandiflorum, J. sambac, J. auriculatum, other spp.*)*

Perfumery: Middle note

There are so many wonderful species and varieties of jasmines to choose from! The scent is sweet, uplifting, and a bit like that of gardenia. A slight resemblance to orange blossom can also be noted. The following scents are characteristic: *J. grandiflorum* (and *officinale*) is sweet, clear, smooth, slightly indolic, iconic white floral. *J. sambac* is spicy, fruity, warm, slightly indolic. *J. auriculatum* is sharp green floral, strongly indolic.

GROWING GUIDELINES

Jasmine vines and shrubs are perennials and thrive in zones 8–11. The plant size can range from dwarf to 30 feet (9 m), and they like full sun or partial shade, moderate water, and well-drained soil. They are very easy to grow. You need a good-size shrub, at least 5 feet (1.5 m) tall and as wide, to begin your processing. Harvesting will be time-consuming but worth it. You will need several full-grown bushes or vines of tiny-flowered jasmine varieties, such as *auriculatum* and *officinale*, to obtain enough for harvesting, and you will need to plan for sequential enfleurage or tincturing or infusing charges.

PREPARATION FOR PERFUMERY

Grandiflorum, officinale, and *auriculatum* are harvested in the morning, before noon. *Sambac* is harvested at night. Sometimes local conditions will change those times, so let your nose be your guide. Carefully remove the flower from the stem, using caution not to bruise the delicate petals. The exception would be "Grand Duke of Tuscany," which will not bruise easily because of its dense cluster of thick petals, but that flower does need to be harvested when 100 percent white. If brown has appeared on the petals, it is decaying. When harvesting, place the flowers in a breathable container, such as an open bowl or bucket, or mesh bag. Quickly process them after only a slight wilt, maybe one hour at most.

PROCESS KEY

	TIME	NOTES
TINCTURE	Level 1. Up to 24 hours, or until saturation	Jasmines are easy to tincture and yield a delightful product. Just opening the jar and inhaling is a wonderful experience. It will take a number of recharges to reach this level of scent, but it's well worth it.
INFUSION	Level 2. **Hot:** 1 hour or less. **Cold:** Several hours to several days	See tincturing notes above. Very easy to infuse, and you'll obtain a fabulous product.
DISTILLATION	Varies according to the distillation method and manufacturer's suggestion	Distillation yields very little oil but a lot of hydrosol.
ENFLEURAGE	Until petals turn translucent, start to brown, or no longer give off scent	All jasmines are highly rewarding enfleurage flowers. Because of their large size, "Grand Duke of Tuscany" *sambac* flowers are good candidates for traditional or large-container enfleurage.

JUNIPER BERRY

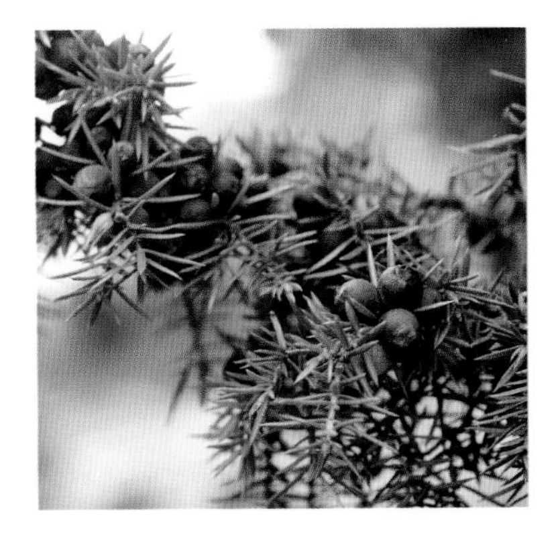

(*Juniperus communis*, other spp.)

Perfumery: Top note

Juniper berries are actually the female cones of this conifer, containing seeds. The berries have a green, warm, fresh, balsamic coniferous scent with some citrus and woody tones. The scent of the essential oil changes dramatically upon dilution to 10 percent or less—people immediately recognize it as "gin," the alcoholic beverage. Juniper berries are the main ingredient in the herbal recipe for gin, but in perfumery, the berries provide a lively top note that blends well with other aromatics. Some species of juniper berries are toxic, so confirm that the plant you are growing or harvesting is of a nontoxic variety.

GROWING GUIDELINES

Juniper has a range of growth that covers zones 2–10, and this perennial can grow from 1 foot to 60 feet (30 cm to 18 m), depending on the species and variety. It likes full sun, but can tolerate some shade, and the water needs depend on the species. It does like moist soil.

Plants give a moderate yield of berries, so you need a good stand of plants for a harvest. If you don't have access to the berries on a wild plant that you have positively identified, it is best to buy the dried berries in bulk from an herb-supply house. Both fresh and dried yield a delightful extract.

PREPARATION FOR PERFUMERY

Juniper berries take two to three years to ripen on the plant, and there will be green berries on the plant at the same time, but do not harvest the green ones. Wait until the juniper berries turn a deep, dark blue color because that signals that they're completely ripe. They may be slightly soft when squeezed. Picking the berries is fairly easy, and slightly drying them will lessen the water weight for distillation.

PROCESS KEY

	TIME	NOTES
TINCTURE	Level 2. May take several days to tincture	Juniper berries do not need to be dried before tincturing, but you can tincture the dried berries if purchased. Crush them for processing.
INFUSION	Level 3. **Hot:** 1 to 2 hours **Cold:** Several weeks	Juniper berries do not need to be dried before tincturing, but you can tincture the dried berries if purchased. Crush them for processing.
DISTILLATION	Varies according to the distillation method and manufacturer's suggestion	Juniper berries are very easy to distill. The oil yield is moderate, and you will get a lot of hydrosol. Crush them for processing.
ENFLEURAGE	N/A	Not a good enfleurage candidate because the berries do not diffuse their scent well.

LABDANUM, CISTUS, ROCKROSE

(*Cistus ladanifer, C. laurifolius, C. creticus,* other spp.)

Perfumery: Cistus essential oil is a top note. Labdanum extracts are base notes.

There are two distinct, different fragrances from one plant: cistus, which is the essential oil distilled from the leaves and flowers, and labdanum, the solvent-extracted resin from the leaves. Cistus: ambery, sweet, balsamic. Labdanum: ambery, musky, deep, balsamic, warm, woody, musky. The showy flowers are very fragrant and come in a variety of colors. Very decorative.

GROWING GUIDELINES

Zones 8 and 9 are best because a zone that is too hot and humid or two cold won't allow this plant to thrive. *C. laurifolius* can be substituted in colder climates. It's an evergreen shrub that varies from dwarf to 8 feet (2.4 m). It likes full sun for resin production, and drought conditions in well-drained soil.

The non-dwarf shrubs are a good size, so one plant should produce enough material for extraction.

PREPARATION FOR PERFUMERY

Hot, sunny weather is the best time to harvest the leaves and flowers from this heat-loving plant. In Crete, temperatures above 85°F (30°C) are regarded as optimum. Cut the flowering branches about 15 inches (38 cm) long, and chop the plant material before processing.

PROCESS KEY

	TIME	NOTES
TINCTURE	Level 1. Up to 24 hours, or until saturation	Cistus tinctures very well and quickly produces a highly scented extract.
INFUSION	Level 2. **Hot:** 1 hour or less. **Cold:** A few hours to a few days	Infusions of cistus yield a lovely oil.
DISTILLATION	Varies according to the distillation method and manufacturer's suggestion	The oil yield is very low, but you'll get a good quantity of hydrosol with a deep base note.
ENFLEURAGE	N/A	Not a good enfleurage candidate because it doesn't diffuse its scent well.
MACERATION IN HOT WATER	Varies	Labdanum is unique in that you can boil the leaves and stems in water and skim off the gummy bits that float, and then mix them with the resin that sinks because it is insoluble in water. An ancient method that is easy for modern perfumers!

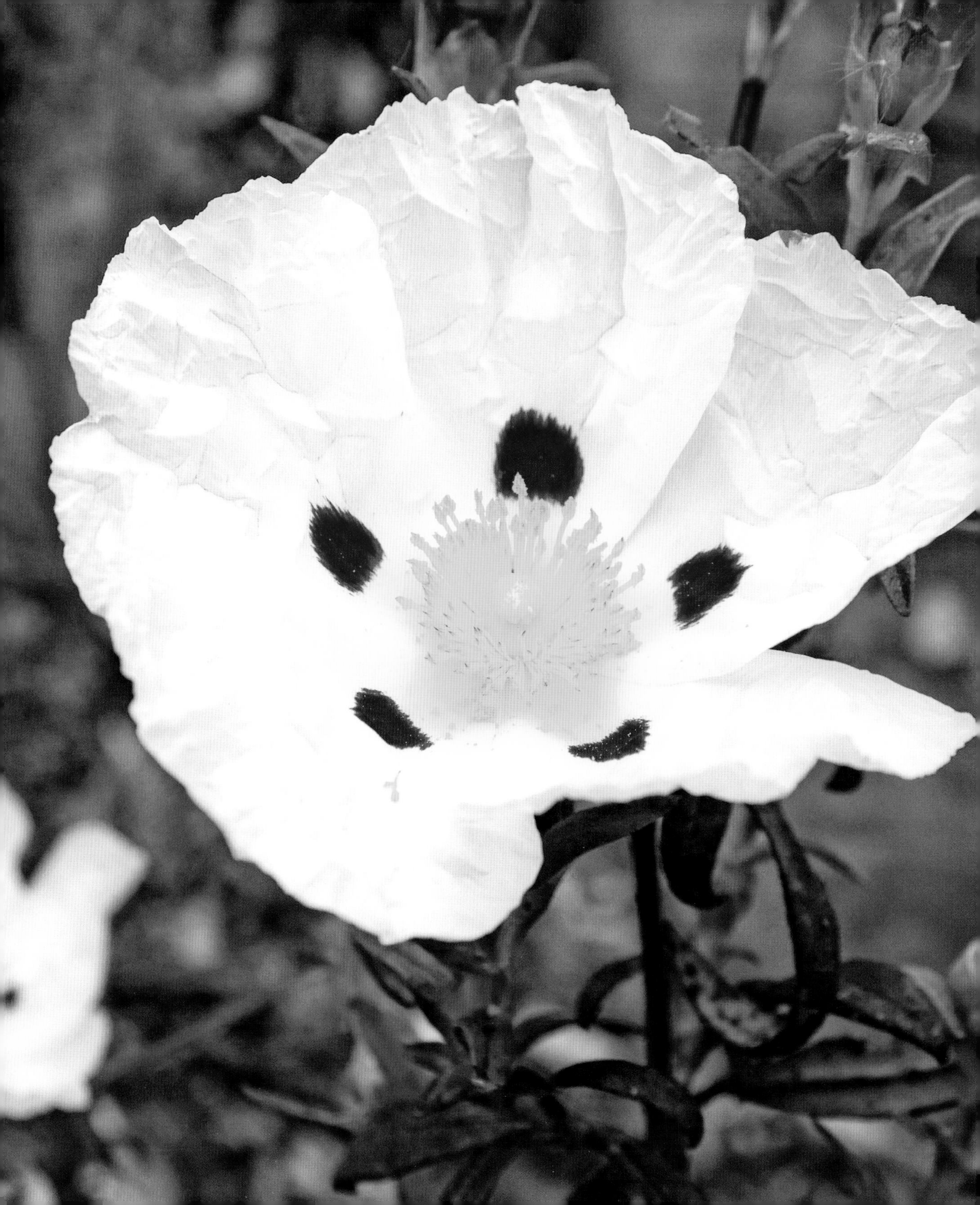

LADY OF THE NIGHT—YESTERDAY, TODAY, AND TOMORROW

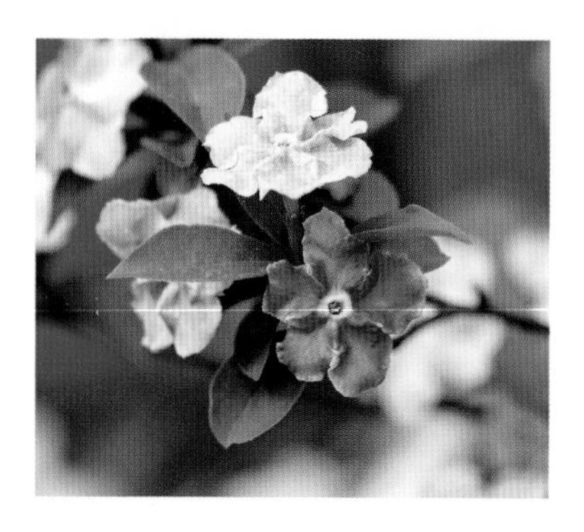

(Brunfelsia grandiflora, B. pauciflora, B. americana, B. lactea, other spp.)

Perfumery: Top to middle note

Different species smell different: The shrubs with the tricolored flowers that are white the first day of bloom, then turn lilac on the second and purple on the third, tend to have a sweet, soft floral scent, much like that of a light gardenia. The species that have white flowers that turn cream are more carnation-like and spicy. On all brunfelsias, the scent becomes strong at night, and they're often scentless during the day.

GROWING GUIDELINES

This perennial group of evergreen shrubs can grow to 12 feet (3.5 m). Partial shade is best, and water requirements can diminish as the plant is established. The plant can be grown as an annual in cold climates, or brought indoors and wintered over, then returned to the garden the next spring. Cuttings root easily for economic reproduction in your garden. The plant is a prolific bloomer, so one large plant, or three to five smaller plants, will provide enough flowers.

PREPARATION FOR PERFUMERY

Pick the fragrant blooms at night, when the scent is the strongest. If you do not want to harvest after dark, you can also experiment with picking them during the day and waiting until nighttime to see whether the scent develops on the harvested flowers. Allow them to wilt for a few hours, if you wish, and then process.

PROCESS KEY

	TIME	NOTES
TINCTURE	Level 1. Up to 24 hours, or until saturation	Tincturing yields a mildly spicy, floral product.
INFUSION	Level 2. **Hot:** 1 hour or less **Cold:** A few hours to a few days	See tincturing notes above.
DISTILLATION	Varies according to the distillation method and manufacturer's suggestion	Distillation can yield a light, refreshing hydrosol but very little oil.
ENFLEURAGE	Until petals turn translucent, start to brown, or no longer give off scent	These flowers may be too fragile for classic enfleurage, but I encourage you to try the large-container enfleurage method, perhaps in a mesh bag, or on a wire cooling rack or a screen, suspended above, but not touching, the fat. Hot enfleurage may be a good option.

LAVENDER

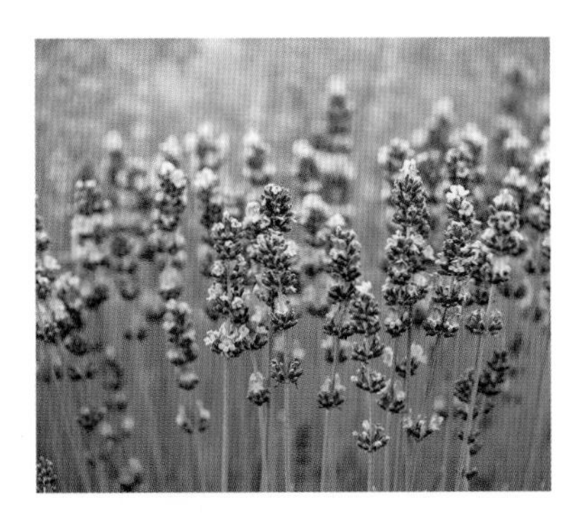

(*Lavandula angustifolia*, other spp.)

Perfumery: Top note/middle note

Lavender flowers are known for their clean, soft, fresh, floral, somewhat antiseptic scent. Scent profiles between the varieties can vary, with sweet and gentle added in for the softer-scented ones, such as *L. angustifolia*, *L. vera*, and *L. officinalis*. *L. stoechas* and other "spike" types are more camphorous, known for their highly antiseptic, sinus-clearing qualities. Most find all lavenders very pleasing and comforting, having had at least some experience with the herbaceous floral, perhaps in the form of soap, an aromatherapy oil, or a body, room, or linen spray.

GROWING GUIDELINES

Lavender is very tolerant of a wide range of growing zones and may produce more fragrant oils on the "fringes" of its recognized zones, which are zones 5–10. It is tolerant of wind, drought, and extreme heat. Most grow to 3 feet (1 m) with similar width.

As few as three or four lavender plants can yield enough flowers in one season to make a highly fragranced quart or liter of infused oil. You may also coax the same quantity of a tincture. If you have room for more, you can grow enough to distill for quality oil and hydrosol.

PREPARATION FOR PERFUMERY

Hot, sunny weather indicates the best time to harvest the leaves and flowers from this heat-loving plant. Cut the flower heads right below where they join the stalk. You can process them fresh or dried or purchase fragrant bunches for your extractions.

PROCESS KEY

	TIME	NOTES
TINCTURE	Level 1. Up to 24 hours, or until saturation	Tincturing lavender is fun because it quickly results in a sweetly floral product.
INFUSION	Level 2. **Hot:** 1 hour or less **Cold:** A few hours to a few days	See tincturing notes above.
DISTILLATION	Varies according to the distillation method and manufacturer's suggestion	Distillation yields a little oil and hydrosol. Fresh lavender distillates (oil and hydrosol) typically do not smell pretty. They must age for a few weeks to several months before they develop their true floral scent.
ENFLEURAGE	N/A	Not a good candidate because it does not diffuse its scent well.

LEMON VERBENA

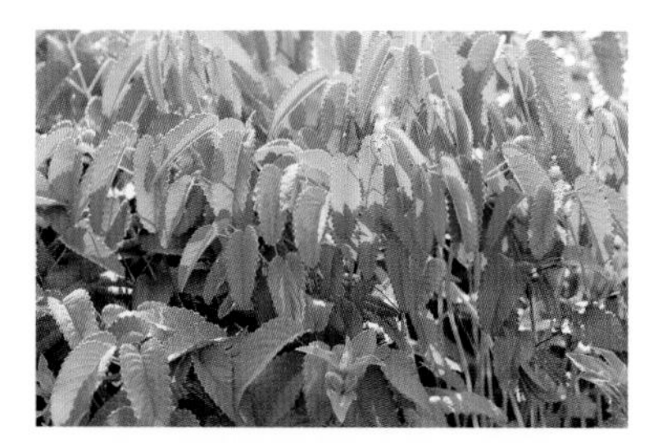

(Lippia citriodora, Aloysia triphylla)

Perfumery: Top note/middle note

Imagine an intensely flavorful, sweet lemon candy—that's the scent of the stiff lemon verbena leaves. It's one of the strongest and clearest lemon scents. The scent persists long after drying, and it smells the same as the day it was picked.

Caution: The essential oil is banned by the European Union as a possible skin sensitizer. Tinctures, infusions, tisanes (teas), and other extractions of lemon verbena are not banned.

GROWING GUIDELINES

This perennial shrub may grow to 6 feet (2 m) or taller in zones 8–10. It likes full sun to partial shade, moderate water (but don't overwater), and well-drained soil. It can be grown in pots in colder climates and brought indoors to overwinter. Cuttings root easily for economical propagation. Seeds are sterile.

One plant should be enough; in a northern climate, you may require three or more. If you plant it in the spring, lemon verbena could produce a good-size shrub by fall, which should provide enough leaves for a project.

PREPARATION FOR PERFUMERY

Harvesting the leaves over the summer will yield enough to make some tinctures or infusions, or additions to recipes. If you have a large shrub in the fall, you may wish to harvest a good part of it for distillation, taking care not to strip the plant or prune it back too severely. Because the leaves dry well and retain their scent for a long time, you can process them at your leisure over the winter. You may also purchase the dried leaves for extraction.

PROCESS KEY

	TIME	NOTES
TINCTURE	Level 1. Up to 24 hours, or until saturation	Tincturing yields a scent that is very true to the plant.
INFUSION	Level 2. **Hot:** 1 hour or less **Cold:** A few hours to a few days	See tincturing notes above.
DISTILLATION	Varies according to the distillation method and manufacturer's suggestion	The plant is notorious for scant oil yield, but it does provide a lot of hydrosol with a rich, bright, fresh scent.
ENFLEURAGE	N/A	Not a good enfleurage candidate because it doesn't diffuse its scent well.

LILAC

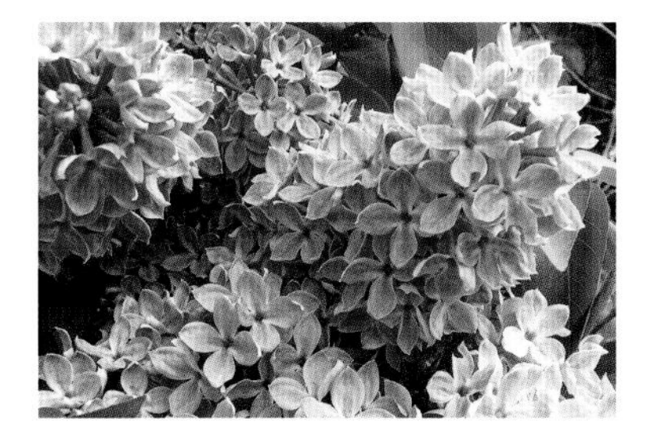

(Syringa vulgaris, other spp.*)*

Perfumery: Top to middle note

The flowers can smell sweet and fresh, then the sweet floral can turn to heavy, the freshness to sultry, and not in a good way. They're somewhat reminiscent of violets and hyacinths, all at the same time, yet they have a unique scent profile. The showy flowers are very fragrant and colors range from white to pink, through lavender, blue, and mauve, to deep purple.

GROWING GUIDELINES

These perennial deciduous shrubs or trees can grow to 10 feet (3 m) in zones 3–7. They need pruning every few years to rejuvenate the plant. Most bloom in spring; some of the new hybrids can bloom into mid- and late summer. They require full sun and a steady supply of water, but do not overwater. One mature shrub can provide enough flowers for several extraction processes or projects.

PREPARATION FOR PERFUMERY

Cut the flowering panicles just as the individual buds begin to open. Process flowers immediately because the top notes dissipate upon wilting or drying.

PROCESS KEY

	TIME	NOTES
TINCTURE	Level 1. Up to 24 hours, or until saturation	Recharge the solvent many times for a strong product. It may take 2 years, given the short flowering season. Refrigerate the tincture to maintain color and scent.
INFUSION	N/A	Not recommended for infusing because the indole is extracted, giving the infusion a rotting smell.
DISTILLATION	N/A	Distillers agree that lilac hydrosol smells terrible. The indole is carried through the steam, but there are no floral notes. No essential oil is produced.
ENFLEURAGE	Until petals turn translucent, start to brown, or no longer give off scent	A very rewarding enfleurage flower, and a good candidate for large-container enfleurage. It's also good for hot enfleurage maceration.

LILY

(Lilium spp.*)*

Perfumery: Middle note

Most lilies share a number of common scents: sweet, heavy floral, slightly spicy, with a touch of vanilla. Each species and variety of lily will smell slightly different. The scent is very diffusive, and a single flower may scent a room. The showy flowers are very fragrant and come in a variety of colors—white, cream, yellow, pink, peach, and crimson. They may be solid or streaked with colors.

GROWING GUIDELINES

Lily flowers grow from bulbs that are perennial and thrive in zones 3–10. Height can range from 1 foot to 6 feet (30 cm to 1 m), depending on type. They like full sun or partial shade, moderate watering, and well-drained soil or the bulbs will rot. They prefer even watering conditions, no drought or flooding. It's hard to predict how many you'll need. Grow as many as you can afford and have space for. That way, you won't overload your extraction container, and you'll have fresh material to recharge the distillation, tincture, infusion, or enfleurage unit.

PREPARATION FOR PERFUMERY

Depending on the type of lily, determine what time of day or night they are most fragrant, and harvest them then. Cut the flower at the top of the stem, where it meets the base of the flower. Avoid crushing or breaking the petals because this can adversely affect the scent, adding unpleasant notes to the extract. Slightly wilt the blossoms before processing them.

Lilies need a lot of room in the extraction container, whether it's a distillation unit, a tincture or infusion container, or an enfleurage container.

NOTE: Lily pollen can be a powerful dye, which may cause your extracts to stain skin and fabric. The pollen can also be poisonous to cats. For a workaround, if your lilies have prominent stamens (the pollen-carrying part at the interior of the flower), hold each blossom upside down and carefully snip off the filament or stems of the stamens before you process the flowers.

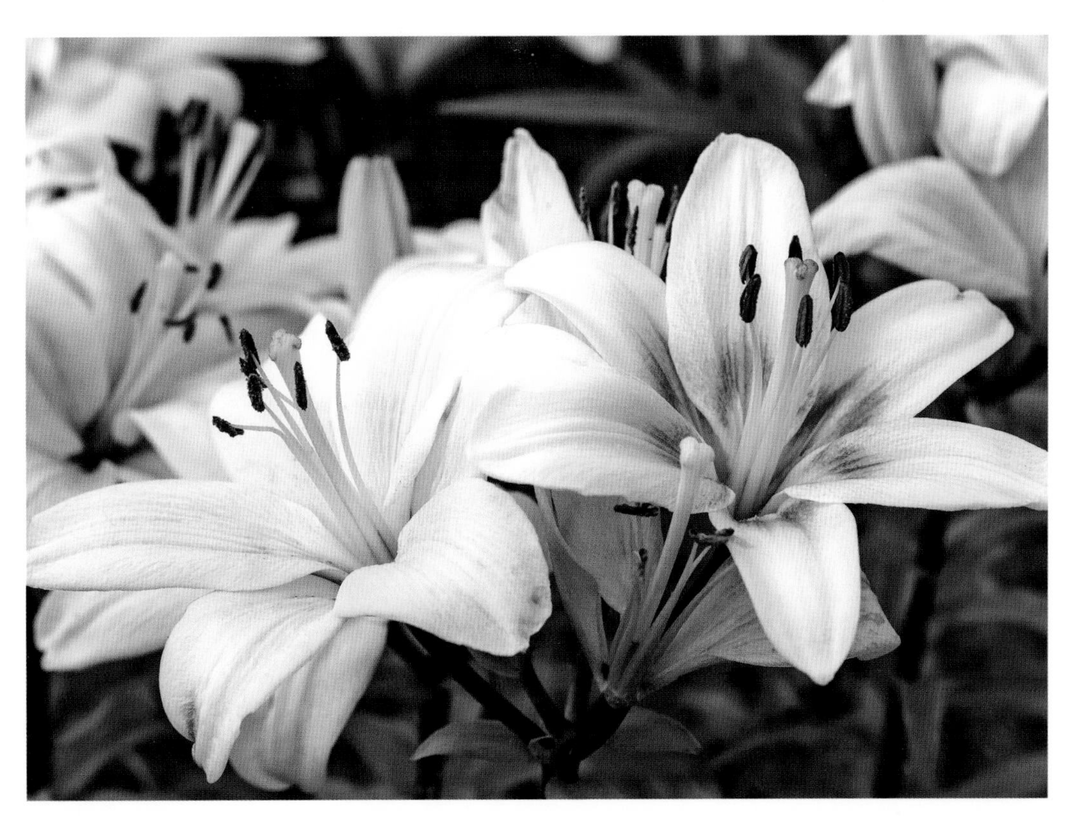

PROCESS KEY		
	TIME	**NOTES**
TINCTURE	Level 1. Up to 24 hours, or until saturation	Requires numerous recharges, resulting in a sweetly floral tincture.
INFUSION	Level 2. **Hot:** 1 hour or less **Cold:** A few hours to a few days	See tincturing notes above. Before infusing, wilt the flowers for 1 to 2 hours to evaporate some of their moisture.
DISTILLATION	Varies according to the distillation method and manufacturer's suggestion	Distillation can be problematic because of the high water content of the lilies. Distillation recharges are not recommended because they can "overcook" the original distillate.
ENFLEURAGE	A few days, several recharges	A very rewarding enfleurage flower, and a great candidate for large-container enfleurage.

LINDEN FLOWER

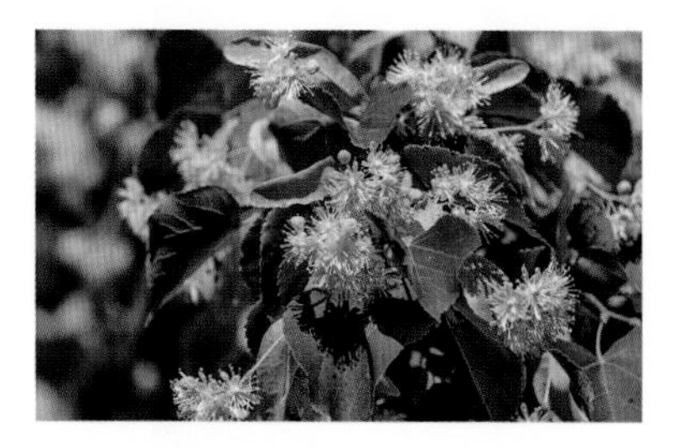

(*Tilia europaea, T. cordata*, other spp.)

Perfumery: Top to middle note

Honey-sweet floral waves of scent envelop someone walking near a linden tree. The flowers fill the air with a tender, beautiful springtime scent. The mild, soothing scent is a favorite for making a floral tea.

GROWING GUIDELINES

The linden tree is best grown in zones 3–8, and it needs a lot of room because it can reach heights of 40 to 130 feet (12 to 39 m). A deciduous perennial, it is often found in parks and lining city streets or grand boulevards. If you have room to grow it on your property, it likes full sun and moderate water; it cannot take a drought. Easy to grow from fresh seeds.

If you have access to one linden tree, you will not lack for material. If you don't have a linden tree on your property, consider searching in your area for one, and then see whether it's possible for you to harvest the flowers. If it's on a city street, you should call the municipality, and ask whether chemicals were used on the tree. Because it is susceptible to insects, it may have been sprayed to control them. You would not want to harvest sprayed flowers.

PREPARATION FOR PERFUMERY

Harvest when the flowers are in full bloom because they're at their full scent potential then. Cut each little flower off at its base. You may choose to dry the flowers for future extraction. The flowers are quite fluffy, so plan for their bulk when you prepare to store them.

PROCESS KEY

	TIME	NOTES
TINCTURE	Level 1. Up to 24 hours, or until saturation	The uplifting scent is easily captured by tincturing. Several recharges are necessary to obtain optimum scent strength.
INFUSION	Level 2. **Hot:** 1 hour or less **Cold:** A few hours to a few days	See tincturing notes above.
DISTILLATION	Varies according to the distillation method and manufacturer's suggestion	Distillation yields little oil but lots of hydrosol.
ENFLEURAGE	Until petals turn translucent, start to brown, or no longer give off scent	Linden flowers are good candidates for large-container enfleurage, with the flowers contained in a mesh bag, or on a wire cooling rack or a screen, suspended above the pomade.

MAGNOLIA, AMERICAN

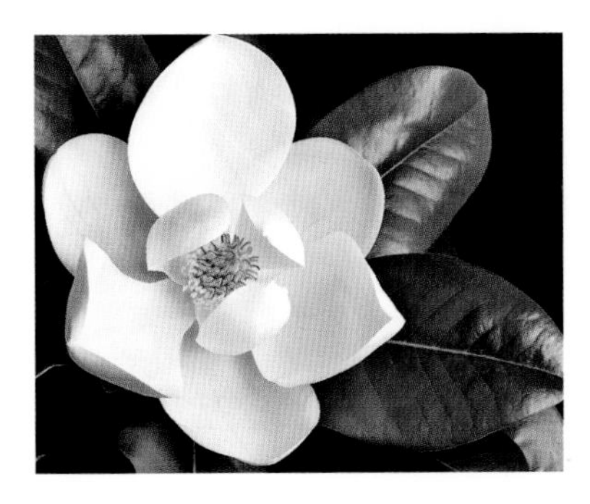

(*Magnolia grandiflora*, other spp.)

Perfumery: Middle note

Most of the magnolia species have the iconic scent of a white, creamy flower. There is, however, a varied scent profile among them, including *M. denudata,* which smells like lemon; *M. hypoleuca,* like ripe melon; and *M. salicifolia,* like lemon and anise. Others have been described as tropical fruit with spice, or a fruit cocktail, with a mélange of fruit scents. The showy flowers are very fragrant, creamy white, and, in some areas, deep pink on the outside of the petals.

GROWING GUIDELINES

These perennial trees and shrubs are evergreen (some are partially deciduous) and grow in zones 6–10. They like full sun but may tolerate partial shade. Provide moderate water, but do not overwater. They are easy to grow and easy to propagate from cuttings. One shrub or tree in bloom will provide many flowers for your extraction purposes—probably more than enough.

PREPARATION FOR PERFUMERY

Harvest the flowers when they are in full bloom, before they begin to decline, which can happen quickly. They do not retain much of the high top notes upon drying. The flowers contain a lot of water, which can be challenging for many extraction methods. Wilt slightly and process quickly.

PROCESS KEY

	TIME	NOTES
TINCTURE	Level 1. Up to 24 hours, or until saturation	Remove the petals from the flowers and slightly wilt them for an hour or so to evaporate some of their water content before tincturing them.
INFUSION	Level 2. **Hot:** 1 hour or less **Cold:** A few hours to a few days	See tincturing notes above.
DISTILLATION	Varies according to the distillation method and manufacturer's suggestion	See tincturing notes above.
ENFLEURAGE	Until petals turn translucent, start to brown, or no longer give off scent	A good candidate for either traditional or large-container enfleurage. Wilt the flowers for an hour or so before placing them on the fat. Flowers can be prepared for enfleurage whole. Pay attention for any sign of mold. This is most easily avoided by changing the flowers daily.

MARIGOLD

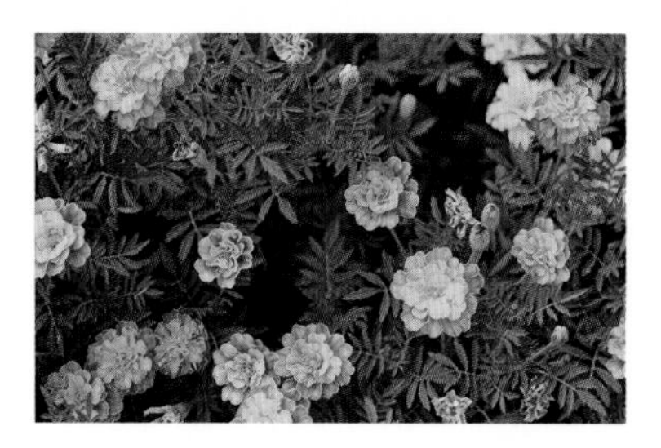

(*Tagetes minuta*, other spp.)

Perfumery: Top to middle note

Marigolds have a fresh, pungent, green, musky scent, which is hay-like, with a hint of apple and herbs. It can be categorized as uplifting and invigorating. Several varieties are grown for perfumery, although *T. minuta* is the most common. All species have slightly different scents. The showy flowers are very fragrant and come in a variety of colors.

GROWING GUIDELINES

Marigolds grow in all zones but the coldest. They are annuals, and are adaptable to most climates, growing in very cold to very hot and humid regions. Single-flowered ones do best in the humid tropics. Heights can vary from 8 to 18 inches (20 to 45 cm) for the French ones, and up to 40 inches (1 m) for the African varieties. They like full sun to partial shade, moderate water, and well-drained soil. They are easily grown from seed.

It takes a few dozen plants to provide enough flowers for your projects. The larger-flowered marigolds are preferred for extraction because they provide the most raw materials.

Multi-petaled (double) ones can quickly provide sufficient materials for extraction from a 12-foot (3.5-m) row. Marigolds dry well, so if you like them a lot, you can grow a large quantity and dry them for future extractions.

PREPARATION FOR PERFUMERY

Harvest when the flowers are in full bloom, before they start to go to seed. You can harvest them any time of day, and they will withstand some wilting while retaining their scent.

PROCESS KEY

	TIME	NOTES
TINCTURE	Level 1. Up to 24 hours, or until saturation	Place the entire flower in the solvent.
INFUSION	Level 2. **Hot:** 1 hour or less **Cold:** A few hours to a few days	See tincturing notes above.
DISTILLATION	Varies according to the distillation method and manufacturer's suggestion	Distillation yields little oil but a lot of hydrosol.
ENFLEURAGE	N/A	Not a good candidate because it doesn't diffuse much, but it can be worth experimenting with large-container enfleurage.

MINT

(*Mentha × piperita* [peppermint], *M. spicata* [spearmint], other spp.)

Perfumery: Top note, used sparingly in fine perfumery, used freely in colognes and body, linen, and room sprays

The leaves of the two most common mints, spearmint and peppermint, smell similar but are distinct from each other. Many people call spearmint the "warm" mint, and peppermint the "cool" mint, which may be due to its high menthol content. Both mints, and the other assorted mints and hybrids, are known for their zesty, fresh, herbal, clean scents.

GROWING GUIDELINES

These perennial plants grow freely in zones 3–11. You may find some types are more adaptable to your area. For example, spearmint does better than peppermint in warm zones. They can grow to 18 inches (45 cm), and they spread by runners. Aerial parts can be harvested ½ inch (1.3 cm) from the soil. Be sure to allow at least one pair of leaves to remain on each stem for repeat growth during the season. May do best in full sun in northern regions and partial shade in the hot, humid South. Most require moisture, but some will survive slight drought. Cuttings root easily for propagation.

Placing a small plant in the soil in springtime can provide a lush bed for harvest by fall. If you are growing several types, separate them as far apart in the garden as you can to avoid hybridization. Cutting off flowering heads before they fully develop also helps prevent hybridization. Mints are "cut and come again" plants during their growing season; pruning makes them bushier.

PREPARATION FOR PERFUMERY

When the plants are mature and in flower, gather the mint in handfuls, and use scissors or shears to cut it off close to the ground. You can wilt the mint before processing because it will retain its scent.

PROCESS KEY

	TIME	NOTES
TINCTURE	Level 1. Up to 24 hours, or until saturation	Mint tinctures rapidly, producing a well-scented tincture in a week or two with only one or two recharges.
INFUSION	Level 2. **Hot:** 1 hour or less **Cold:** A few hours to a few days	See tincturing notes above.
DISTILLATION	Varies according to the distillation method and manufacturer's suggestion	Distillation yields some oil and a lot of hydrosol.
ENFLEURAGE	N/A	Mints are traditionally not suited to enfleurage because they do not diffuse their scent.

NARCISSUS, JONQUIL, DAFFODIL

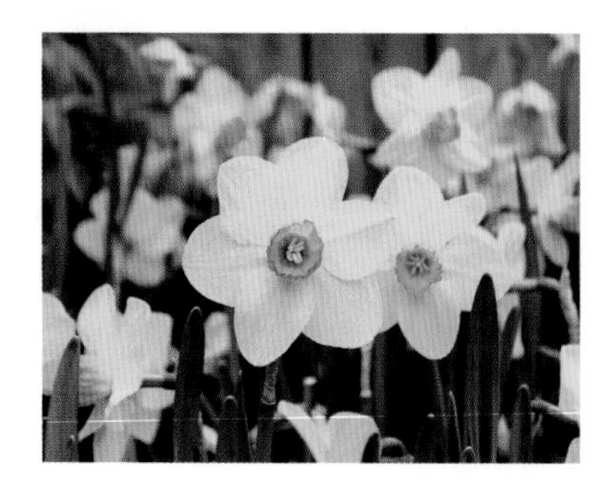

(*Narcissus poeticus, N. jonquilla*, other spp.)

Perfumery: Middle note

Most narcissi are airy, spicy-floral, slightly green. A soft, deep, liquor-like floral note, smooth and rich, with a touch of carnation, describes its close relative, the jonquil. The other important narcissus is the daffodil, which has a fresh, spring-like scent—a bright and cheerful floral. There are single- or double-flowered types in colors ranging from white to peach, yellow, orange, red, apricot, and cream or off-white.

GROWING GUIDELINES

If you don't have a garden space for them, narcissus "paper white" bulbs can be purchased in the fall and will bloom indoors. Jonquils and daffodils require fall planting of the bulbs to give them a chilling period for the flowers to develop. You can "force" the bulbs by storing them in the refrigerator. Planting them in the ground allows them to naturalize and spread in subsequent years, increasing your yield. The bulb supplier will have specific instructions for their successful growth. They do best in colder climates, zones 3–8. They'll grow to about 18 inches (45 cm). Full sun to partial shade, constant watering, and well-drained soil are necessary. Ask your local garden centers, local USDA service center, or Master Gardeners to determine which cultivars are most fragrant in your locale.

Each bulb produces a minimum of one to three flowers; a few dozen flowers will fill an enfleurage tray. Enfleurage is the traditional method of extraction, and recharges are necessary to obtain a strong-scented product. If you already have a stand of narcissi, jonquils, or daffodils, you will have a sufficient amount for the first year. If not, you can plant the bulbs in the fall and look forward to them multiplying in coming years.

PREPARATION FOR PERFUMERY

Your nose will tell you when the flowers reach full fragrance. Pick them the first day of fragrant bloom to optimize your harvest. Snip the flower just under the bloom with scissors. Try to process them immediately, or after a slight wilting.

PROCESS KEY		
	TIME	**NOTES**
TINCTURE	Level 1. Up to 24 hours, or until saturation	The solvent needs numerous recharges for a strong-scented product. Refrigerate this delicate tincture until use.
INFUSION	Level 2. **Hot:** 1 hour or less **Cold:** A few hours to a few days	Many people prefer this method because it is reputed to extract the freshest scent. The flowers need to be wilted first to remove excess moisture. See tincturing notes above.
DISTILLATION	Varies according to the distillation method and manufacturer's suggestion	You may obtain a delicately scented hydrosol, and a tiny amount of oil.
ENFLEURAGE	Until petals turn translucent, start to brown, or no longer give off scent	All narcissus spp. flowers are wonderful candidates for either traditional or large-container enfleurage.

NIGHT-SCENTED STOCK

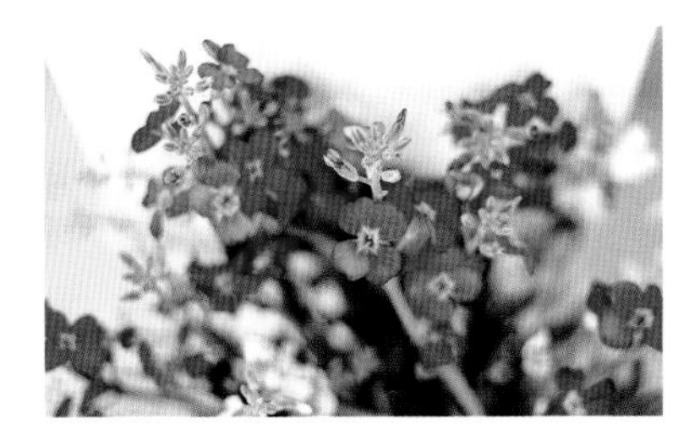

(Matthiola bicornis, M. longipetala)

Perfumery: Middle note

The fragrance of night-scented stock is sweet, intoxicating, heady, vanilla, musky, floral, and cinnamon/clove/carnation spicy. The white, rose, and lilac-colored flowers may appear limp during the day, but they refresh in appearance and pump out their fragrance at dusk.

GROWING GUIDELINES

Gardeners debate whether the *longipetala* species has a stronger scent than the *bicornis*, but they are often sold without proper identification, so purchase seeds from a reputable dealer, grow both, and decide for yourself. The nighttime perfume from these little plants wafts for a great distance, and is beloved by many people because of its beauty. It will grow from zones 1 to 11 and is very hardy and dependable. It will grow to 18 inches (45 cm) in full sun to partial shade, with moderate water. Do not allow to dry out.

If you grow about 50 plants, you will have more than enough for several extractions. I have filled up an enfleurage tray with the eight or so stalks that I purchased in a grocery store for a reasonable price.

PREPARATION FOR PERFUMERY

You'll want to harvest the fully open flower stalks at night, when the scent is strongest, by cutting the stem just beneath the stalk. You can remove the individual flowers from the stalk because you do not want to process the stalk if you distill, tincture, or infuse. The stalk may be left on for enfleurage. Work quickly, and do not allow the flowers to wilt.

PROCESS KEY

	TIME	NOTES
TINCTURE	Level 1. Up to 24 hours, or until saturation	Requires many recharges to obtain a strong tincture.
INFUSION	Level 2. **Hot:** 1 hour or less **Cold:** A few hours to a few days	See tincturing notes above.
DISTILLATION	Varies according to the distillation method and manufacturer's suggestion	It should be hydro-distilled with gentle heat and low pressure. Distillation yields very little oil but a lot of hydrosol.
ENFLEURAGE	A few days, several recharges	A very rewarding enfleurage flower. It's a good candidate for either traditional or large-container enfleurage, as well as hot enfleurage maceration.

PALMAROSA

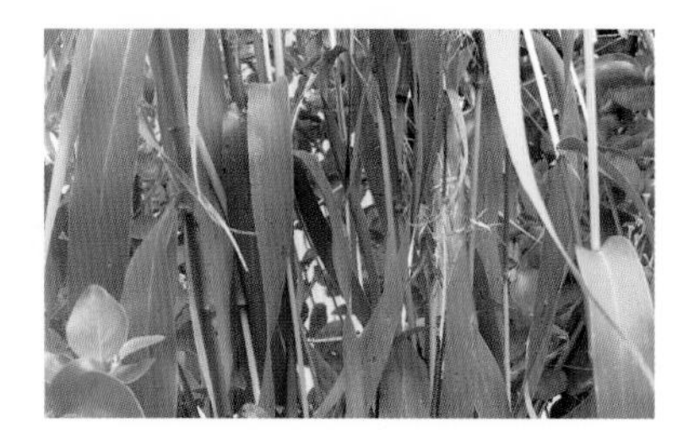

(Cymbopogon martinii var. *motia)*

Perfumery: Top to middle note

This grass plant is highly aromatic with a floral aroma of citrus and rose.

GROWING GUIDELINES

Palmarosa is a tropical plant and will grow outdoors in zones 10–11. It's easy to grow in pots, so it can be brought indoors during cold weather. This perennial can grow to 9 feet (3 m), will resprout from the roots after cuttings, and will yield essential oil for several years. It is not attractive, so don't feature it in a prominent spot in the garden. Needs full sun to bright shade; water to establish, but water sparingly after that.

Three to four plants will provide enough material for extraction. The grass and flowers both contain the essential oil. Palmarosa is a quick growing, spreading grass, and at the end of one growing season, you should have a large amount of leaves and flowers to harvest. They dry well, so what you don't extract at harvest you can use later.

PREPARATION FOR PERFUMERY

The grass can be harvested just as it matures and puts out flowers. To reduce moisture in processing, I recommend drying the plant for a day or two before processing it.

PROCESS KEY

	TIME	NOTES
TINCTURE	Level 1. Up to 24 hours, or until saturation	Chop the leaves into small pieces, about 2 inches (5 cm) long for tincturing.
INFUSION	Level 2. **Hot:** 1 hour or less **Cold:** A few hours to a few days	See tincturing notes above.
DISTILLATION	Varies according to the distillation method and manufacturer's suggestion	Distillation yields a small quantity of oil and a richly scented hydrosol.
ENFLEURAGE	N/A	Palmarosa is not a candidate for enfleurage because it does not diffuse its scent well.

PEONY

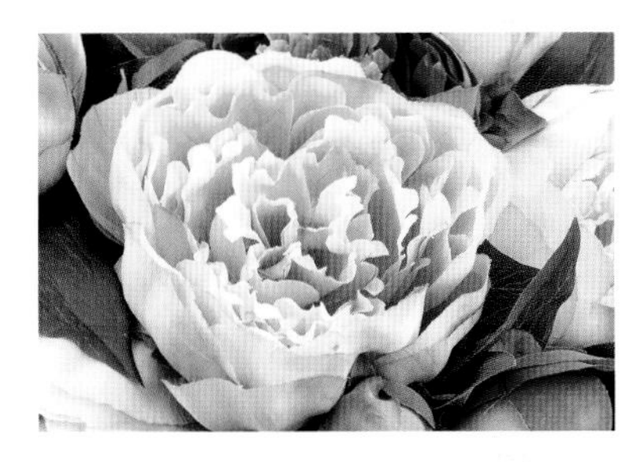

(*Paeonia* spp.)

Perfumery: Middle note

The fragrant peonies have a range of scents, from a beautiful, delicate rose-like fragrance to a lemony, and even ginger-like, spice scent. Large, "fluffy" (many ruffled) petals make the peony flower a beautiful garden asset. They come in beautiful colors, from white, peach, and cream through medium pink.

GROWING GUIDELINES

These perennial shrubs grow well in zones 4–8 and do not grow in hot or humid areas. They reach a height of 3 to 5 feet (91 cm to 1.5 m) and like full sun or partial shade. Water sparingly. One large shrub of peonies will provide you with a substantial amount of flowers to work with.

PREPARATION FOR PERFUMERY

Harvest the blooms in the spring, just as the flower begins to open. Work quickly because the blooming season is short, and, if possible, find varieties that may extend the bloom time. The fragrance will last a few days, but process them before they wilt.

PROCESS KEY

	TIME	NOTES
TINCTURE	Level 1. Up to 24 hours, or until saturation	Requires many recharges to obtain a strong-scented tincture.
INFUSION	Level 2. **Hot:** 1 hour or less **Cold:** A few hours to a few days	See tincturing notes above.
DISTILLATION	Varies according to the distillation method and manufacturer's suggestion	Distillation yields very little oil but a lot of hydrosol.
ENFLEURAGE	Until petals turn translucent, start to brown, or no longer give off scent	A very rewarding enfleurage flower. A good candidate for large-container enfleurage.

ROSE

(*Rosa × centifolia, R. × damascena, R. moschata*, other spp.)

Perfumery: Middle note

Mention the word roses and people have a scent memory of a floral, pleasant aroma. The fragrance can vary from fresh, green, musky, spicy, citrusy, and at least a dozen other scent descriptors. You can process both fresh flowers from your garden and dried rosebuds from a supplier. The fresh flowers will give you a light "rose water" type of product, and the dried buds provide a deeper, warmer scent.

GROWING GUIDELINES

Choice of variety to grow can vary by zone, and they grow in zones 2–11. Check with local nurseries, and ask whether a specific rootstock is needed in your area. They can come in many forms: ground cover, trained, standard, shrub, or climbing plant. Full sun to partial shade, with at least six hours of sun a day. Don't allow the plants to sit in water or dry out; they like the middle ground regarding moisture. Prevent water from splashing up on the leaves to prevent diseases.

Rosebush yields can vary greatly according to the variety; plan on one to five bushes to start with. With a modest harvest, several recharges of a tincture or infusion can provide a usable product that you can add to over time. Most small distillation units hold 2 liters of material for one distillation.

PREPARATION FOR PERFUMERY

Pick the blooms when they are half to fully open in late morning, after the morning dew is gone, and before the heat of the day evaporates the essential oil from the petals.

Be careful not to crush or otherwise damage the flowers because this leads to quick decomposition. Do not place them in a plastic bag or container where moisture may build up. Instead, use a basket or cloth bag.

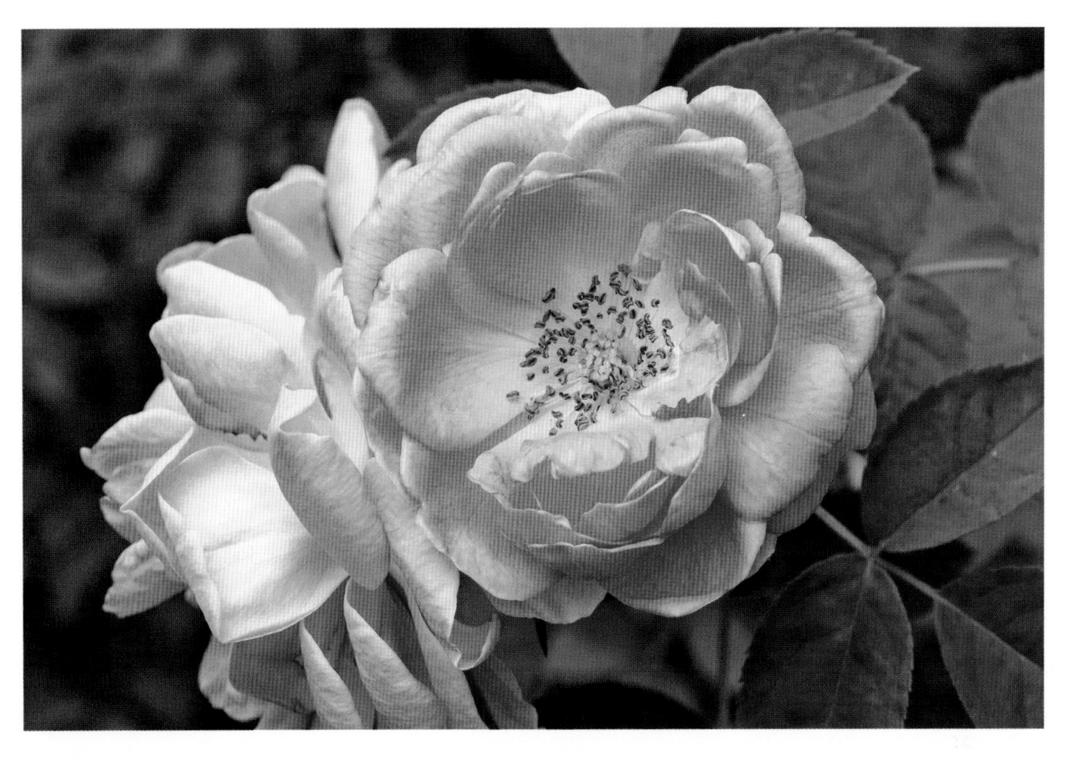

PROCESS KEY		
	TIME	**NOTES**
TINCTURE	Level 1. Up to 24 hours, or until saturation	Tincturing roses is highly rewarding; a strong tincture results from charging a half dozen times or less. Dried roses swell in the solvent. If you're using dried material, use a wide-mouth jar and check to see whether more solvent is needed after initial absorption.
INFUSION	Level 2. **Hot:** 1 hour or less **Cold:** A few hours to a few days	See tincturing notes above.
DISTILLATION	Varies according to the distillation method and manufacturer's suggestion	Distillation yields very little oil but a lot of hydrosol. Rose petals are best hydro-distilled, rather than steam distilled, because steam distillation can cause them to clump and scorch.
ENFLEURAGE	Until petals turn translucent, start to brown, or no longer give off scent	For traditional enfleurage, use only sturdy, large-petaled roses, and gently open the petals, placing them side-by-side. Remove the petals after one day and recharge with fresh ones. Smaller, more delicate roses, as well as large, cabbage-type ones, are good candidates for large-container enfleurage. Roses are also great for hot enfleurage maceration.

ROSEMARY

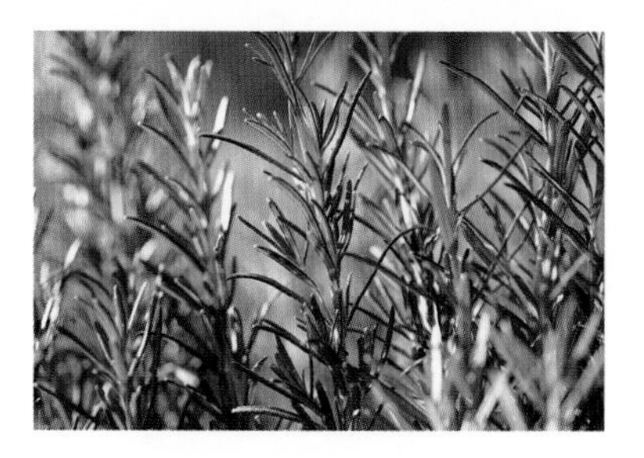

(Rosmarinus officinalis)

Perfumery: Top to middle note

Rosemary leaves have a strong odor that is very herbaceous and terpenic, reminiscent of pine needles. Some varieties may be sharply camphorous, clearing your sinuses. Others are softer and most suited for food, beverages, and perfumery. The soft-scented ones are recommended for perfumery.

GROWING GUIDELINES

Rosemary is a perennial and grows best in zones 7–10. It likes full sun with moderate water, just to establish the plant. It can take drought conditions after that. Varieties come in sizes ranging from a low ground cover to a tall shrub, up to 6 feet (2 m) tall. Easy to grow in pots and move indoors in cold climates.

If you grow *R. officinalis* or one of the many large-growing types of rosemary, in one year you'll have a huge plant, and you can take many cuttings. Grow more than one, and you'll be sure to have a good supply for many extraction projects.

PREPARATION FOR PERFUMERY

It is economical to buy small plants and let them grow out for one season. The growth will be slow at first, but the plant will fill out and surprise you with the size it can reach by fall. In milder climates, it will continue to grow year-round. The branch tips can be clipped throughout the growing season for use in scent extraction. For extracting scent, you may also include the flowers in the clippings.

PROCESS KEY

	TIME	NOTES
TINCTURE	Level 1. Up to 24 hours, or until saturation	Rosemary is easy to tincture, releasing its scent rapidly into the solvent.
INFUSION	Level 2. **Hot:** A few hours **Cold:** Several weeks	See tincturing notes above.
DISTILLATION	Varies according to the distillation method and manufacturer's suggestion	Decide which scented rosemary you like, and distill that variety. Distillation yields very little oil but a lot of hydrosol.
ENFLEURAGE	N/A	Rosemary is not a good candidate for enfleurage because it does not diffuse its scent well.

SWEET WOODRUFF

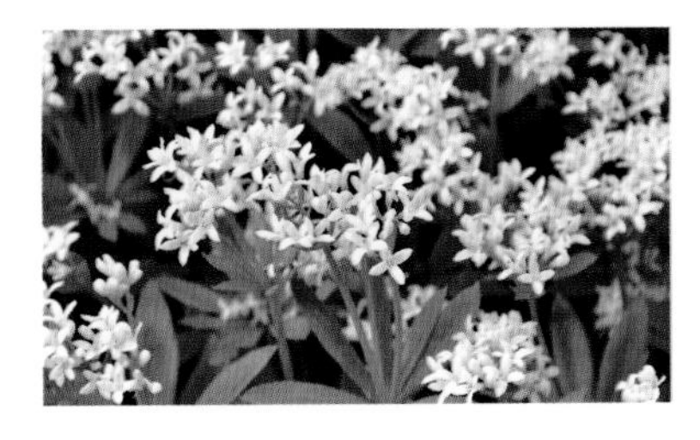

(Galium odoratum, Asperula odorata)

Perfumery: Middle to base note

The entire plant smells like vanilla and new-mown hay, which is the grassy scent associated with coumarin, a vanilla, hay-like aroma. Very pleasing, soft, gourmand fragrance. Scent is most prominent in understory growth, perhaps a bit wilted and brown.

GROWING GUIDELINES

Grows best in zones 4–8, where it will receive a chilling, dormant period in winter. This pretty plant with white flowers is a spreading ground cover, up to 12 inches (30 cm) high. Needs partial to deep shade; sun will kill it. Heavy irrigation is needed if there is a dry spell, as it requires a lot of water. It is easily propagated by root divisions. A good ground cover, densely planted at least 10 feet (3 m) by 10 feet (3 m), will supply the gardener with a steady supply. Do not clear-cut the area—just selectively thin out plants.

PREPARATION FOR PERFUMERY

Cut it near the base, taking care not to uproot the plant. Harvest the entire plant, snipping the foliage and flowers an inch (2.5 cm) or more above the soil. Allow some foliage so the plant can regenerate. Include some of the dried, older material on the ground if you are going to extract it for perfumery. The more dried material, the better.

PROCESS KEY

	TIME	NOTES
TINCTURE	Level 2. Several hours to several days	Sweet woodruff tinctures very easily, yielding a strong-scented product.
INFUSION	Level 3. **Hot:** 1 hour or less **Cold:** A few hours to a few days or weeks	See tincturing notes above.
DISTILLATION	Varies according to the distillation method and manufacturer's suggestion	Distillation yields very little oil but a lightly scented hydrosol.
ENFLEURAGE	N/A	Not a good candidate for enfleurage because the scent does not diffuse well.

TOBACCO, FLOWERING

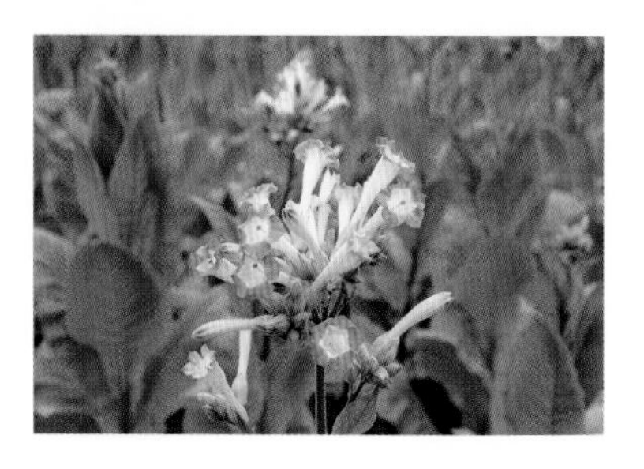

(Nicotiana alata)

Perfumery: Middle note

There is a spicy carnation-like note that carries the flowering tobacco scent far from the planting bed. It smells like a touch of clove and has a soft floral aspect that is enticing. The sticky hairs on the flowers will transfer their scent to your hands.

GROWING GUIDELINES

Flowering tobacco grows in zones 6–11 and may be a perennial in warm climates. In colder zones, replant it annually. It grows from 18 to 36 inches (45 to 90 cm). The flowers are fragrant at night, and the white-flowered varieties have the strongest scent. It takes full sun or partial shade and likes moist soil conditions. Make sure you don't buy the scentless hybrids.

A garden row or plot with at least 50 plants should provide enough flowers for a one-season harvest. Flowering tobacco plants are succession bloomers, which means as you remove blooms, more will grow from side shoots.

PREPARATION FOR PERFUMERY

Cut the flowers where they join the stem. Cut at night when they are the most fragrant. If you need to cut them when it is still daylight, experiment with the variety you have and see whether they develop scent after the sun goes down. If so, you can process them as if they were cut at night.

PROCESS KEY		
	TIME	**NOTES**
TINCTURE	Level 1. Up to 24 hours, or until saturation	Should be used only in products that are not applied to skin, such as room and linen sprays.
INFUSION	N/A	Not recommended because of potential skin irritation.
DISTILLATION	Varies according to the distillation method and manufacturer's suggestion	Not a good candidate for distillation because there is very little oil, and the hydrosol scent may dissipate quickly. Spray on fabric or use as a room spray.
ENFLEURAGE	Until petals turn translucent, start to brown, or no longer give off scent	Flowering tobacco is a good subject for both traditional and large-container enfleurage. The pomade is good for use in hair dressing, but should not be worn on skin.

TUBEROSE

(Polianthes tuberose)

Perfumery: Top to middle note

The reputation of the strong scent of the "narcotic" white flowers has been the stuff of legends. The sultry, intense, and spellbinding white flower scent is like no other, although some comparison is made to gardenia. A single stalk in bloom can fragrance a room with its heady, sweet, and sexy perfume. It is a heavy, creamy, white floral; exotic, rich, sweet, wine-like, diffusive, cloying, and dark, with a touch of decay. It reveals its scent at night.

GROWING GUIDELINES

Tuberose flower stalks grow from a bulb, and it does well in zones 8–10, except for zone 10 in Florida because of soil nematodes. You can grow it in containers, and it's best to purchase forced bulbs each season, or force them yourself. It's a perennial, typically growing to 2 feet (60 cm). It flowers best in full sun and likes moderate water and well-drained soil. It takes many flowers to produce a strong extract. I recommend starting with 50 to 100 bulbs.

PREPARATION FOR PERFUMERY

The fully developed bud, about to open, is harvested for enfleurage. If open, you may still use it for enfleurage, but it is best saved for distillation or tincturing at that point. Harvest the flower buds by carefully removing them from the stem. I have used open flowers for tincturing, distilling, and large-container enfleurage. Wait until night to harvest so you have the most fragrant ones. They should be processed immediately and not allowed to dry out.

PROCESS KEY

	TIME	NOTES
TINCTURE	Level 1. Up to 24 hours, or until saturation	Tuberose can be tinctured, but it is almost a waste of the flower because submerging it in alcohol halts the scent release, which otherwise can continue for days.
INFUSION	Level 2. **Hot:** 1 hour or less **Cold:** A few hours to a few days	The infusion will be inferior in scent to tincture, distillate, and pomade. In addition, the flowers are susceptible to rotting in the oil.
DISTILLATION	Varies according to the distillation method and manufacturer's suggestion	Distillation yields very little oil but a lot of hydrosol.
ENFLEURAGE	Until petals turn translucent, start to brown, or no longer give off scent	An exceptional candidate for traditional enfleurage. Unopened or slightly opened buds are best because the life span of the scent dispersal is longer than with flowers that are already open.

VETIVER

(Vetiveria zizanioides, Chrysopogon zizanioides)

Perfumery: Base note

The aromatic, dried roots of vetiver smell earthy, woody, sweet, green, rich, musty, dry, bitter, ambery, salty, and balsamic. Yes, all of those contradictory terms describe vetiver because it is a very complex aromatic. The scent of the oil is very strong and very long-lasting.

GROWING GUIDELINES

Vetiver grows in zones 8–11 and can take a light freeze in colder areas. This perennial grass has fragrant roots that grow very deep, up to 20 feet (6 m), but you can grow it successfully in a deep, wide pot. Don't try to grow it in the ground, as digging the roots out will be quite tedious and nearly impossible. A good-size pot would be 2 to 3 feet (0.5 to 1 m) tall and 3 feet (1 m) wide, or larger. It takes 18 months for the roots to mature from a tiny plant. It likes full to partial sun and needs regular water in the pot. Potting soil will need to be washed off once the roots are harvested. It is easily propagated for the next season from a small side cutting with some root attached. For the beginner, just one tiny plant in a large pot will give you a huge harvest of dense but lightweight roots in 18 months.

You may also buy dried vetiver from online sources. It is quite "fluffy" or bulky. One pound (454 g) is sufficient for several processes.

PREPARATION FOR PERFUMERY

I was the first artisan perfumer to grow vetiver in the United States for scent extraction. Here are my results from trial-and-error growing, harvesting, and processing it.

The roots are best harvested at 18 to 24 months of age. When the plant is ready to harvest, allow the soil to dry out a bit, turn the pots on their side, and pull the plant out by the grassy foliage. Then cut the foliage off and begin to beat the soil from the roots with a board or pipe, turning the root-ball frequently. I always finish cleaning the roots with jet streams of water from the hose. I like to do this by setting the roots on an open-weave chair or table so that the good soil from the root-ball washes down and is returned to the ground. Cleaning the vetiver is quite challenging, but the yield is great, so it's worth it. After confirming there is no more soil, you can dry the root-ball by hanging it in a dark, dry place. After it is dry, pull the root-ball apart into usable bunches and store them in airtight containers. To prepare the roots for extraction, pound them a bit with a rubber mallet or hammer to break open the cells for easier access to the scent molecules. You can also chop them up, either in addition to or in place of pounding.

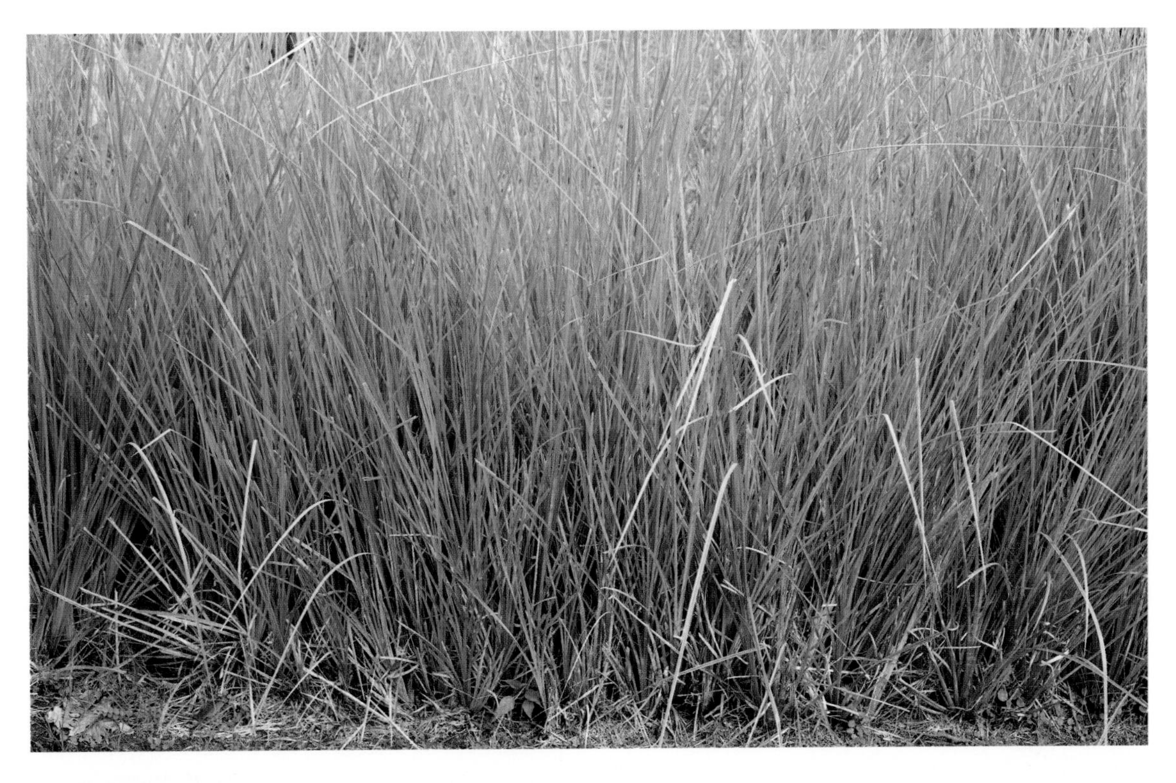

PROCESS KEY		
	TIME	**NOTES**
TINCTURE	Level 3. 1 to 2 weeks, and can be left in the tincture indefinitely	Lends itself very well to tincturing. It tinctures rapidly and efficiently, giving a quick, rewarding product for your perfumes. Chop the roots to aid the process.
INFUSION	Level 3. **Hot:** 2 hours or less **Cold:** A few weeks	See tincturing notes above. Hot infusing is most effective. Yields a strong infusion that is good for oil or solid perfumes and for massage or hair oils.
DISTILLATION	Varies according to the distillation method and manufacturer's suggestion	Hydro-distillation is recommended. Distillation yields more oil than most plants and a lot of hydrosol. Soak the dried roots in water for 1 day before distillation. You can also chop them into 2-inch (5-cm) pieces.
ENFLEURAGE	N/A	Not a good candidate for enfleurage because it does not diffuse its scent well.

YLANG-YLANG

(Cananga odorata var. *genuina)*

Also: Dwarf ylang-ylang *Cananga fruticosa;* ylang-ylang vine *Artabotrys hexapetalus.*

Perfumery: Middle to base note

The flowers have an intensely sweet, tropical, rich, and floral scent with hints of fruit and spice. There may also be a slightly balsamic, richly green note, especially in the extracts. It is called the "Chanel No. 5 tree" because it is an important ingredient in that perfume. There are two smaller options for the perfume gardener to grow: dwarf *Cananga*, and the *Artabotrys* vine. Both have scent similar to the *C. odorata* tree.

GROWING GUIDELINES

This perennial tropical tree does well in zones 10 and 11. The trees are relatively easy to grow; they like full sun and moderate water. Irrigate if leaves droop. Heights of various ylangs: *C. odorata:* 60-foot (18-m) woody evergreen tree; *C. fruticosa:* shrub up to 6 feet (2 m); A. hexapetalus vine: 18 feet (5.5 m). If the smaller varieties are grown indoors, high humidity must be maintained, or leaves will turn black and die. Because a tree can dwarf a home garden, I do what the growers do in Madagascar to make the flowers easy to harvest—I have it pruned to keep it about 6 feet (2 m) tall. It makes a squat-looking tree because the branches are about 6 feet (2 m) long, with big, drooping leaves, sort of like a large, square hedge. One productive tree may provide enough flowers for several extractions over a long season.

PREPARATION FOR PERFUMERY

The flowers are light green when just budding and turn a rich yellow with a red center when ready for harvest. Harvest them first thing in the morning, or when the aroma is strongest. The most fragrant ones waft their scent closest to midnight. I wear a headlamp and beekeeper's netting hat so that I can see the flowers and keep the bugs away from my face. Ylang-ylang often blooms year-round. Flowers can be harvested throughout the bloom cycle, and they have different scents from the green to fully yellow stage. So if the scent of the green ones still maturing appeals to you, use them. However, the fully ripened bright yellow flowers with the touch of red in the center are the most desirable, having the strongest, most developed scent.

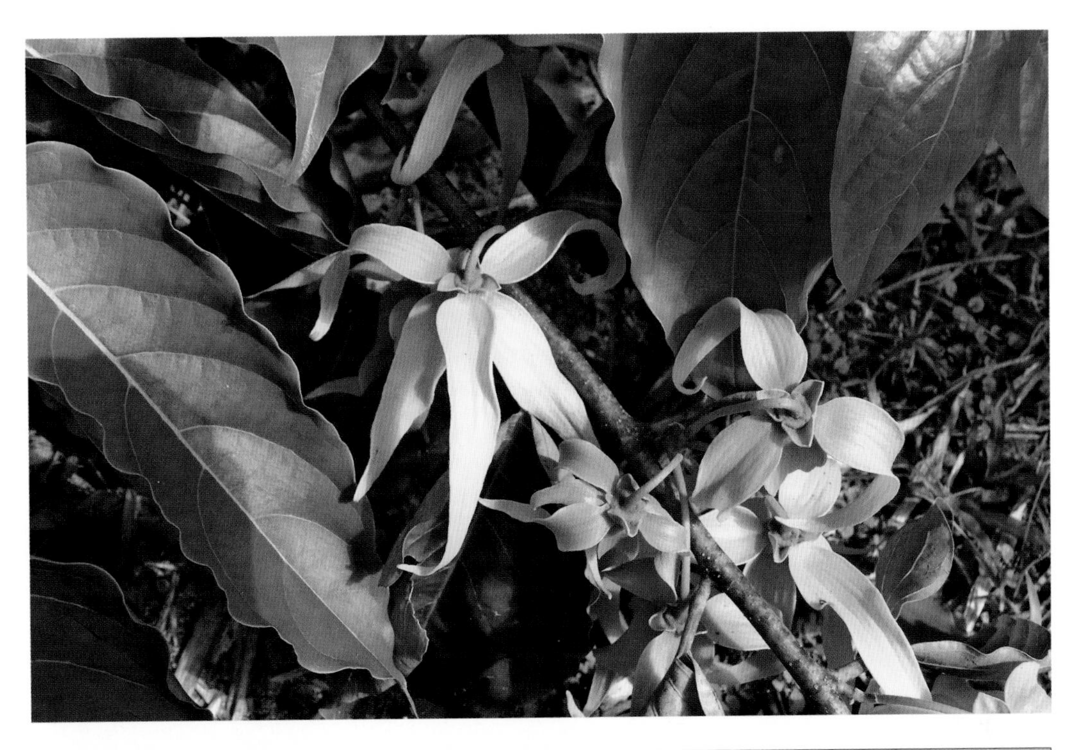

PROCESS KEY		
	TIME	**NOTES**
TINCTURE	Level 1. Up to 24 hours, or until saturation	Very easy to tincture, producing a strong-scented extract that is long-lasting.
INFUSION	Level 2. **Hot:** 1 hour or less **Cold:** A few hours to a few days	See tincturing notes above.
DISTILLATION	Up to 15 hours for the various stages of scent extraction; much less if distilling for a "complete" version of oil	The flowers are water distilled or water and steam distilled over many hours. One kilogram of flowers can yield 20 milliliters of essential oil, making it one of the most productive perfume flowers. Research further to discover specific distillation times for specific fractions (extra, I, II, and III), and for ylang-ylang complete.
ENFLEURAGE	Until petals turn translucent, start to brown, or no longer give off scent	Ylang-ylang is not traditionally used for enfleurage because the flowers rapidly fall apart and decay. However, large-container and powder enfleurage are perfect extraction methods for this good-sized flower. Use a mesh bag or other perforated container to hold them, and watch closely for signs of decay.

OTHER FRAGRANT PLANTS THAT YOU MAY WISH TO GROW

There are thousands of fragrant plants, and you may have some that aren't in this book, or you may decide to research further and see if you want to include these in your garden. If you identify the flower, leaf, wood, or root type as close to the texture described in the Levels Method Timetable on page 32, experiment and see if you can extract the scent with one of the methods. Have fun!

- Adam's needle *(Yucca filamentosa)*
- Almond bush *(Aloysia virgata)*
- Apple blossom *(Malus pumila)*
- Black locust *(Robinia pseudoacacia)*
- Boronia *(Boronia megastigma)*
- Boxwood (*Buxus* sp.)
- Camellia × 'High Fragrance,' other spp.
- Carissa *(Carissa grandiflora)*
- Chinese perfume tree *(Aglaia odorata)*
- Clematis *(Clematis odorata)*
- David's clematis *(Clematis davidiana)*
- Day lily (*Hemerocallis aurantiaca,* other spp.)
- Dittany *(Dictamnus fraxinella)*
- Dracena, corn plant *(Dracaena fragrans)*
- Easter lily vine *(Beaumontia grandiflora)*
- Egyptian blue lotus *(Nymphaea caerulea)*
- Evening primrose *(Oenothera caespitosa)*
- Fragrant mountain azalea *(Azalea canescens)*
- Freesia (*Freesia grandiflora,* other spp.)
- German iris (*Iris germanica,* other spp.)
- Golden currant *(Ribes aureum, R. odoratum)*
- Heliotrope *(Heliotropium arborescens)*
- Herbaceous clematis *(Clematis recta)*
- Honey locust (*Gleditsia triacanthos,* other spp.)
- Lavender (*Lavandula vera,* other spp.)
- Lemon beebalm *(Monarda citriodora)*
- Lemongrass *(Cymbopogon citratus, C. flexuosus)*
- Mayflower, trailing arbutus *(Epigaea repens)*
- Mock orange (*Philadelphus coronarius,* other spp.)
- Monarda (*Monarda* spp.)
- Musk mallow *(Malva moschata)*
- Night-blooming cereus *(Epiphyllum oxypetalum)*

- Night-blooming jasmine *(Cestrum nocturnum)*
- Osmanthus *(Osmanthus fragrans)*
- Pear blossom (*Pyrus communis*, other spp.)
- Phlox (*Phlox paniculata*, other spp.)
- Pink shower tree *(Cassia nodosa)*
- Privet *(Ligustrum ovalifolium)*
- Pua keni keni *(Fagraea berteriana)*
- Rhododendron, azalea (*Azalea viscosum*, other spp.)
- Rose daphne (*Daphne cneorum*, other spp.)
- Sacred or Indian lotus (*Nelumbo nucifera*, other spp.)
- Scented geraniums (*Pelargonium*, other spp.)
- Scotch pink *(Dianthus plumarius)*
- Siberian flowering crabapple *(Malus coronaria)*
- Southernwood *(Artemisia lactiflora)*
- Spike winter hazel *(Corylopsis spicata)*
- Strawberry shrub *(Calycanthus floridus)*
- Sweet acacia, mimosa (*Acacia farnesiana*, other spp.)
- Sweet pea *(Lathyrus odoratus)*
- Sweet pepperbush *(Clethra alnifolia)*
- Sweet sultan *(Amberboa moschata)*
- Thimbleberry *(Rubus odoratus)*
- Viburnum (*Viburnum*, other spp.)
- Wallflower *(Cheiranthus cheiri)*
- Western catalpa *(Catalpa speciosa)*
- White clover (*Trifolium repens*, other spp.)
- Witch hazel *(Hamamelis virginiana)*

APPENDICES

APPENDIX 1: USDA PLANT HARDINESS ZONES

The current map of the United States Department of Agriculture (USDA) plant hardiness zones is fairly intricate, containing 26 specific climatic designations for the continental United States, Alaska, Hawaii, and Puerto Rico. The zones have changed over the years, and if you've lived in the same place for many years, you most likely find your zone warmer than it used to be.

You can call your local USDA Cooperative Extension to confirm your zone. I recommend establishing a relationship with them to learn more about the possible microclimates on your property. This can help you to decide where to grow your plants. The following link to the updated USDA zone map allows you to enter your zip code to find what your current zone is: planthardiness.ars.usda.gov.

APPENDIX 2: SOURCING ALCOHOL

The supplier list in Appendix 3 gives several sources for alcohol in the United States. The most readily available nonorganic alcohol is Everclear, a grain alcohol that is available in both 151 and 190 proof at most liquor stores.

Some states strictly regulate the sale of alcohol, and some ban the sale of 190-proof alcohol. There are online stores that can get around this for the most part, but you need to check your state's laws. The online stores cannot ship to some states, and they list them on their websites. I have heard of people driving to the next state to buy their supply for perfumes, or having friends or relatives bring it to them, so that may be an option for people in states that prohibit 190-proof alcohol. However, I'm not condoning violating the law, merely passing along what I've learned.

Shipping and hazmat (hazardous materials) fees add a lot to the cost of high-proof alcohol. The current 2018 price of 190-proof Everclear is about $16 (USD) per liter. There may be an additional $30 shipping/hazmat fee if you have it shipped to you. Organic alcohol costs around $115 (USD) per gallon, with a $40 shipping/hazmat fee. The shipping fee is higher the farther you are from the shipper. Some online sites recommend that you buy 3 liters at once so that you can save on the fees because they are combined in one order.

APPENDIX 3: SUPPLIERS AND REFERENCE WEBSITES

I list only suppliers that I have had direct buying experience with and that sell high-quality materials. I encourage you to obtain samples from numerous suppliers and compare them first, and then buy larger quantities based on your comparison. This can save you time and money rather than obtaining aromatics that aren't of the quality or specific scent you expected.

Alcohol (undenatured 190-proof ethanol)	A Web search is the best way to locate Everclear and other brands of 190-proof ethanol. Everclear is grain alcohol (usually corn) and is not organic. Available by mail order in some states; inquire whether you can have it delivered in your state. **Alchemical Solutions:** Organic corn, sugar, and grape alcohol http://organicalcohol.com
Beeswax	I recommend the granules for ease of use. Search the Web or eBay for white (decolorized) or golden beeswax granules.
Bottles and jars for perfumes, sprays, and body care	Visit the following websites, or Amazon and eBay, to see if they have bottles and jars to fit your needs. Some sites are wholesale with high minimums, but most are retail. Try to source near you because glass can be heavy and costly to ship. You can also search for vintage bottles and jars on eBay. **ABA Packaging:** http://abapackaging.com **Accessories for Fragrances:** http://accessoriesforfragrances.com **Acme Vial:** http://www.acmevial.com **Alice-Aliya:** http://www.alicealiya.com **E.D. Luce Packaging:** http://essentialsupplies.com **Madina Industrial Corporation:** http://madinaonline.com **Nemat International:** http://www.nematinternational.com **New High Glass:** http://newhighglass.net/#!/container/Home **Perfume Trade Worlds:** http://perfume.tradeworlds.com/web_category_4842.html **Pilot Vials:** http://www.pilotvials.com **Save on Scents:** http://www.saveonscents.com/index.php/cPath/1 **Sunburst Bottle:** http://www.sunburstbottle.com **True Essence:** http://www.trueessence.com/bottles-packaging/
Butters and waxes	Search the Internet, eBay, and Amazon.

(continued)

Calculators, online, for dilutions, percentages, volumes, weights	http://www.math.com/everyone/calculators/calc_source/percent.htm http://percentagecalculator.info/ http://www.math.com/students/calculators/source/3percent.htm
Distillation units/stills	**The Essential Oil Company:** http://essentialoil.com **Copperstills:** http://www.copperstills.com **HeartMagic:** http://heartmagic.com eBay and Amazon are good sources for other distillation units; especially small, beginner sizes.
Dried woods and resins	**Apothecary's Garden:** https://apothecarysgarden.com/ **Mermade Magickal Arts:** http://www.mermadearts.com **Scents of Earth:** http://www.scents-of-earth.com/index.html See also Incense warmers for vapor and smoke enfleurage (below).
Enamel or stainless steel trays	Search the Internet, eBay, thrift stores, and garage sales.
Essential oils and absolutes	Suppliers at http://naturalperfumers.com. Check as more vetted suppliers are added to this list on the website. **Av-At:** http://www.av-at.com **Arlys Naturals:** http://www.arlysnaturals.com **Cherry Valley Lilacs:** http://cherryvalleylilacs.com **Eden Botanicals:** http://www.edenbotanicals.com **Enfleurage:** http://www.enfleurage.com **Essential Oil Co.:** http://www.essentialoil.com **The Lermond Company:** http://lermond.com **Timeless Essential Oils:** http://timelessessentialoils.com Other suppliers: **Aromatics International:** http://aromaticsinternational.com **Liberty Natural:** http://libertynatural.com **Nature's Gift:** http://naturesgift.com **White Lotus Aromatics:** http://whitelotusaromatics.com

FDA Good Manufacturing Practices (GMP)	http://www.fda.gov/cosmetics/guidanceregulation/guidancedocuments/ucm353046.htm Links to this page change every few years. If this link does not work, search the Internet for FDA GMP.
Filter papers	Coffee filters can work for most projects. **Orlandi USA:** http://orland-usa.com Various online retailers
Fresh fragrant flowers	**Hawaii:** http://www.mauifloral.com **New York City:** http://gpage.com Search online for wholesale flower suppliers to purchase aromatic plants such as gardenia and tuberose. Currently, online wholesale prices are really high. Find local suppliers, if possible, to avoid high shipping costs. Ask for "seconds"—flowers that are not aesthetically perfect for the retail market—because these are more affordable. I've bought three gardenia seconds for $6.
Herbs and spices	**Mountain Rose Herbs:** http://mountainroseherbal.com **Penn Herb Co.:** http://pennherb.com **Penzeys Spices:** http://penzeys.com
Incense warmers for vapor and smoke enfleurage	**Mermade Magickal Arts:** http://www.mermadearts.com
Jars for tincturing, infusing, and storage	I recommend using canning jars; they can be found in many supermarkets, hardware stores, and even thrift shops.
Laboratory equipment	I find beakers, filter paper, graduated cylinders, and pipettes on eBay and Amazon.
Natural Perfumery Yahoo! group	https://groups.yahoo.com/neo/groups/NaturalPerfumery/info
Non-hydrogenated vegetable shortening	Many supermarkets and health food stores carry this; also available as organic.

(continued)

Nurseries for fragrant plants	It's always nice to find plants locally, but if you can't, I highly recommend these sources: http://companionplants.com http://logees.com http://rareflora.com http://toptropicals.com http://whiteflowerfarm.com **Scented geraniums (Pelargoniums)** http://www.accentsforhomeandgarden.com http://geraniaceae.com/cgi-bin/viewCat.py?c=Pelargoniums (Scented Leaf Section) **Tuberose bulbs** http://tntuberoses.com
Oils for infusions	Internet, local health food stores, and co-ops
Presses for tinctures, infusions, and hot enfleurage	Simple tincture and herb presses or potato ricers can be found on eBay and Amazon and at retail stores and thrift shops. Plans to build a simple herb press: http://practicalprimitive.com/skillofthemonth/tincturepress.html Detailed plans to build a hydraulic press for oil enfleurage: http://curezone.com/forums/fm.asp?i=1865771#i
Suet and lard for traditional enfleurage	Fannie and Flo have these supplies: https://www.etsy.com/shop/FannieAndFlo?ref=l2-shopheader-name Check local butchers to obtain these materials for enfleurage. If none is available locally, search the Internet for sources that ship.
Testing laboratories	**Essential oils testing:** Laboratoire PhytoChemia: http://www.phytochemia.com **Hydrosol testing:** Superior Labs, Inc. superiorlabs@aol.com

ACKNOWLEDGMENTS

Brian Michael Shea, Paula Diaz, Andrea Abbott Ganuza, Gracie Kahlo Reyes, Ana Trusty, Adrian Jai Denuzzo, Jimmy, Michael Orkin, Daniella Vargas, and Gabriela Serra, thank you for your help with the garden, the perfume business, and for your companionship on the many fragrant projects.

To my parents, for encouraging reading and education. To my brother William J. McCoy III for being a steady, loving force in my life. To the lovely, nurturing Cedella Marley Booker, thank you for being a mom to me.

Bruce Bolmes and Michael Singels, I appreciate your help with technical, chemical, and mathematical assistance on many projects .

Christine Ziegler, Catherine Symonds, and Andrine Olson, you are sisters in the natural perfumery world, and the decades of friendship, sharing, and laughs are forever in my heart. Bob McCulley, your memory lives on as a gardening expert and friend.

Frode Wells, my computer life could not be so steady and productive without your years of help with any problem, and hours of garden chat while things got fixed.

Robert Tisserand, you are a delight to confer with, and my first inspiration in the aromatherapy world with your first book *The Art of Aromatherapy*. Jeanne Rose, your book *Herbs and Things* awakened my senses to so much botanical beauty, and Mindy Green, you are a delight and a beacon in the world of herbs and aromatherapy; thank you for your advice. Chrissie Wildwood, I adored our chats and I love your aromatherapy books; thank you so much for all you have done.

Christina Dickson, Robyn McKeithan, Amy Elaine Abrams, Estella Garcia, and Harry Kutcher, thank you for extending my family circle. Gabrielle Howard, you help keep the house and studio together with humor and delight.

Julia Onnie-Hay, an herbalist close to my heart, you are building the South Florida herb community. Eugene A. Anderson, PhD, my economic botany professor, thank you for encouraging me to develop my own major at UCRiverside. Valerie Pantanelli, your physical therapy helped me walk so much better; I appreciate it. John A. Starnes, your advice about growing roses in Florida has been invaluable, and inspired me to start growing these beautiful flowers again. Dr. Robert Zablotowicz, "Zap," thank you for your indulgence of me, just out of my teens, on my quest for fragrant plants, aromatic oils, and the study of perfumery; you are missed. Author Diana Rodgers generously forwarded my book idea on to Page Street Publishing, a true gift of fellowship to a stranger, and I am grateful.

Thanks to Page Street Publishing Company for being open to the idea of a book on fragrance and their support and encouragement. My editor Sarah Monroe was the guiding force regarding the direction and organization, and I have much gratitude for her patience.

ABOUT THE AUTHOR

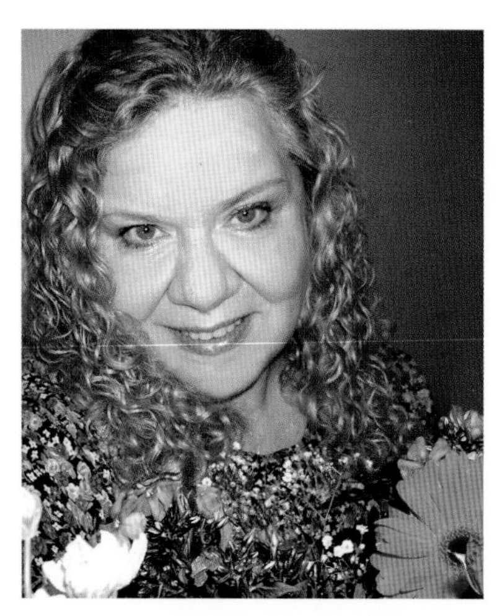

As the perfumer of Anya's Garden Perfumes, Anya McCoy is a pioneer in natural perfumery worldwide. She is the founder and head instructor of the Natural Perfumery Institute, the first online school for natural perfumery, established in 2007. She created a line of natural perfumes in 1991, and subsequently was admitted to the American Society of Perfumers, the first artisan perfumer given this honor. In 1990, she was elected to a State of Florida position as the Soil and Water Conservation District Manager in Collier County. In 2002, she launched a natural perfumery group on Yahoo, which remains the largest repository of information on natural perfumery on the Internet. She is the president of the Natural Perfumers Guild, an international association devoted to natural aromatics. She has won numerous awards for her perfumes, and is always developing modern techniques to enhance the ancient art of natural perfumery. An herbalist, botanist, and aromatherapist, she combines these disciplines in perfumery and frequently blogs about them. Her previous book, *Basic Natural Perfumery* (2010), was the first American textbook on the subject. She has a B.A. in economic botany from the University of California, Riverside, and a master's in landscape architecture from the University of New York, Syracuse. She is a former adjunct professor of urban planning and design at Florida Atlantic University, Fort Lauderdale.

INDEX